WHOLE HEALTH

Simply

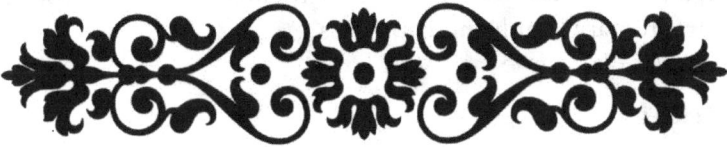

Your Guide to a Life of Extraordinary
Health and Happiness

Margot Dargaville, R.N., I.N.H.C.

This book is dedicated to my family and friends. Thank you for the friendship, love and understanding you have shown me always.

This book is also dedicated to you, on your journey to a lifetime of wellness. May your family and friends travel with you in extraordinary health and happiness.

Margot

Whole Health Simply
Your Guide to a Life of Extraordinary Health and Happiness

Copyright © 2016 by Margot Dargaville

For information, contact Margot Dargaville at

www.wholehealthsimply.com

978-0-9944724-0-3

Printed in Australia

Contents

Introduction

Good health has always been the mainstay of my life. I've been a Registered Nurse, working in hospitals and general practices for many years, and I've spent a lot of time with some very sick people.

They have often become unwell due to the choices made throughout the years, at times without knowledge or understanding of the detriment to their health and well-being. A poor diet, using drugs or alcohol, extended periods of extreme stress, not getting enough exercise or even something as simple as the lack of sunshine can have a hugely negative impact on health.

At times, illness and disease can come into our lives without reason. Helping your body to recuperate can only be supported by giving it the care and nourishment it needs and deserves.

My aim is to help as many people as I can get on track with their diet and lifestyle, and become their healthiest, most vibrant selves.

Life can be tough. And busy. I've been there too.

Motherhood started for me with the diagnosis of a melanoma when our first child was born, and then continued with seemingly endless family dramas - bowel obstruction, asthma attacks and head injuries, to name just a few. I wondered if any of us were going to make it through.

Years of anxiety, and the exhaustion of adrenal fatigue came hand in hand with the stresses of life, and I have made countless, distracted attempts to find a remedy.

Curiosity, a medical background, and a strong desire to know the truth of things, led me to years of constant studying of the most up-to-date health concepts.

I joined the *Institute of Integrative Nutrition* and studied to become a *Certified Health Coach* so that I could work with people and empower them to keep themselves healthy.

Health coaching gave me the inspiration and extra knowledge I needed to make changes in my own life. My efforts have brought me to this place, and I can truthfully say that I'm a much happier, more relaxed, and nourished person.

It's so easy to live your life on autopilot, and not take time to care for yourself properly or listen to your body, especially when you are so busy caring for all those around you.

The good news is that our bodies have an innate ability to repair themselves. All you need is a strategy that's easy to understand and follow through.

The information out there is confusing. I've been through most of it in my quest for solutions.

I wanted to provide an up-to-date, concise, basic prescription for life that I could share with my family and friends. To help them stay energetic, healthy and happy for the rest of their long lives.

This book is the result of my desire to share what I've learned. It will help you live your dreams, and the most beautiful life you can imagine.

Follow the simple daily practices of nourishing your body inside and out, and cherishing yourself and your emotional wellbeing.

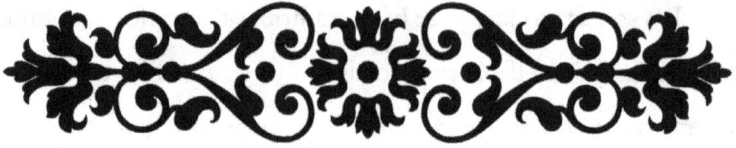

A Basic Prescription
for Lifelong Health and Happiness

The world we live in is an amazing place full of all sorts of technologies like space travel and the internet, and there will still be many changes ahead! We've come so far in so many ways. Technology and our knowledge in some areas are phenomenal.

And yet, we're struggling with this modern world, and the chronic health conditions that have appeared alongside it: autoimmune diseases, cancer, obesity, anxiety, depression and diabetes, to name just a few.

Has technology moved too fast and left us behind? Are we equipped for this modern life, and its constant computer access, artificial lighting, processed foods and sedentary, isolated lifestyle?

For those of us affected by these extremes, we need to build our resilience and recover our health.

This book clearly sets out what you can do each day to set you back on the path to resiliency, and empower you to live your most extraordinarily healthy, happy, and vibrant life.

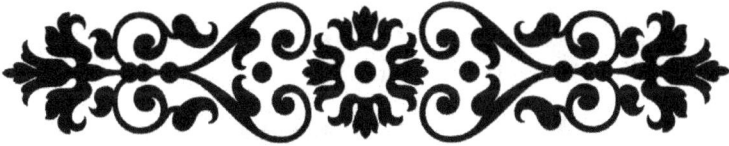

Obesity rates are rising, with 63% of Australian adults at last count being either overweight or obese.[i]

The most common, long-term health conditions in 2012 were arthritis (at 14.8% of the population, that's equal to 3.3 million people), mental and behavioural conditions like depression and anxiety (13.6%), asthma (10.2%) and heart disease (4.7%).[ii] Close to 1 million people in Australia suffer from some form of long-term diabetes.[iii]

The World Health Organisation (WHO) reveals in its 2014 World Cancer Report, how the number of new diagnoses of cancer were growing at an *alarming pace*, with cancer rates in 2012 at 14 million, and expected to rise to 22 million in 2035.[iv]

Health conditions such as asthma, eczema, hay fever, food allergies, lupus, and multiple sclerosis are also on the rise. The incidence of autoimmune disease has quadrupled in the last few decades.[v]

Modern medicine relies on expensive and often potentially dangerous drugs to 'fix' a patient's health, which may only mask the disease by treating the symptoms and not the cause.

By the time the average adult is over 65, they are diagnosed with several chronic conditions - the most common being hypertension, diabetes, osteoporosis, osteoarthritis and chronic lung disease, requiring quite a handful of medications every day for treatment.

Then there are all the other chronic conditions that often worsen with age such as GORD (reflux), depression, anxiety, insomnia, kidney disease, heart disease, and hormonal issues. These are all treated with more medications, which do quite a good job of improving symptoms, but come with their own issues. Side effects and even life-threatening adverse reactions are relatively commonplace.

As the old saying goes – "An ounce of prevention is worth a pound of cure!"

Your body was designed to be healthy without requiring anything more than what it needs to thrive and restore itself. Nourishment in the form of the right foods and a healthy lifestyle…

With family and friends experiencing various forms of modern chronic disease, I have been driven to study dietary and lifestyle changes that are known to have hugely beneficial effects.

Having been a nurse for 38 years, mainly in hospitals and general practice, I followed Western Medicine's path unquestioningly, relying heavily on pharmaceuticals to 'cure' whatever ails us. Unfortunately, the drugs often only serve to improve symptoms of disease, and **don't repair the disease itself.**

Only in recent years have we started connecting the dots.

We are brought up to eat whatever tastes good, let life happen, struggle with chronic disease, and never put the cause and effect together.

One of the goals of this book is to keep you out of hospitals for anything other than emergency and trauma care, which is where our medical system works brilliantly.

You can take control of your health and keep it safe in your own two hands!

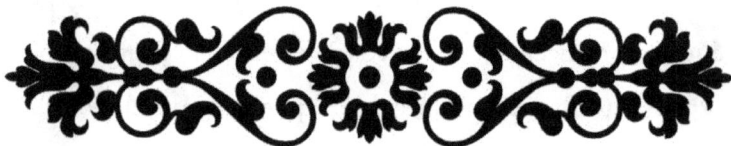

Epigenetics - The New Science

Our DNA has been refined and perfected over millions of years to provide us with optimal health, function and longevity. DNA is organised into genes, and gives your body instructions, like a blueprint, for everything it needs to grow, develop, repair and live well.

The new science of epigenetics has made it clear that where once we believed we were the victims of our family heredity, our genes aren't set in concrete. They are moulded by their environment (your body), and the chemistry of your blood can change the biology and fate of the cells that lie within it.

With this new understanding we know our lifestyle choices - our diet, supplements, exercise, and particularly the emotional content of our daily experiences, all contribute to the chemical reactions within our genes.

Even our day-to-day thoughts and feelings play a huge

role in either disease formation or wellness promotion. This means that the choices we make will activate or deactivate the parts of our genes which code for health OR disease! **It's our choice!**

By being more conscious in the way we live our lives, we can mindfully ensure that our family history will not become our personal destiny.

Epigenetic science has shown that we can change the chemistry of our blood by eating well and maintaining a positive mindset. [vi]

We CAN take charge of our own future!

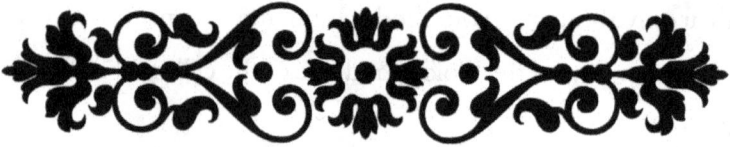

Bio-Individuality

It's important to recognise that each of us is an individual, with individual needs. The centuries old maxim "One person's food is another person's poison" is so true! None of us have exactly the same genetic code. How could any fad diet or restrictive diet work for everyone? It can't, just as there is not one lifestyle that would make everyone happy and fulfilled.

Learn to listen to your body and adjust how you care for it based on the feedback it gives.

Stay focused on the positive changes you want, and not on the things you are trying to avoid.

Approach these changes with curiosity and a sense of adventure. You are sure to enjoy the results!

This book will guide you through the simple actions you can take to make the best choices in diet and lifestyle. Your body is designed to heal itself and, given proper nutrition and care, it will do what it does best and regenerate to its optimal self.

Start with small simple changes. As you read, choose one or two areas to work on at a time and mark them off as you go.

A sample awesome daily routine is included at the back of the book to give you a vision for your future, along with some pages for note-taking.

Design your own awesome daily routine and keep this book with you for inspiration.

Take charge of your future – nourish yourself inside and out. And while you are at it, remember to take care of your emotional wellbeing too!

Happy Reading!

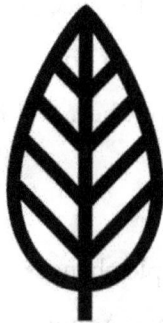

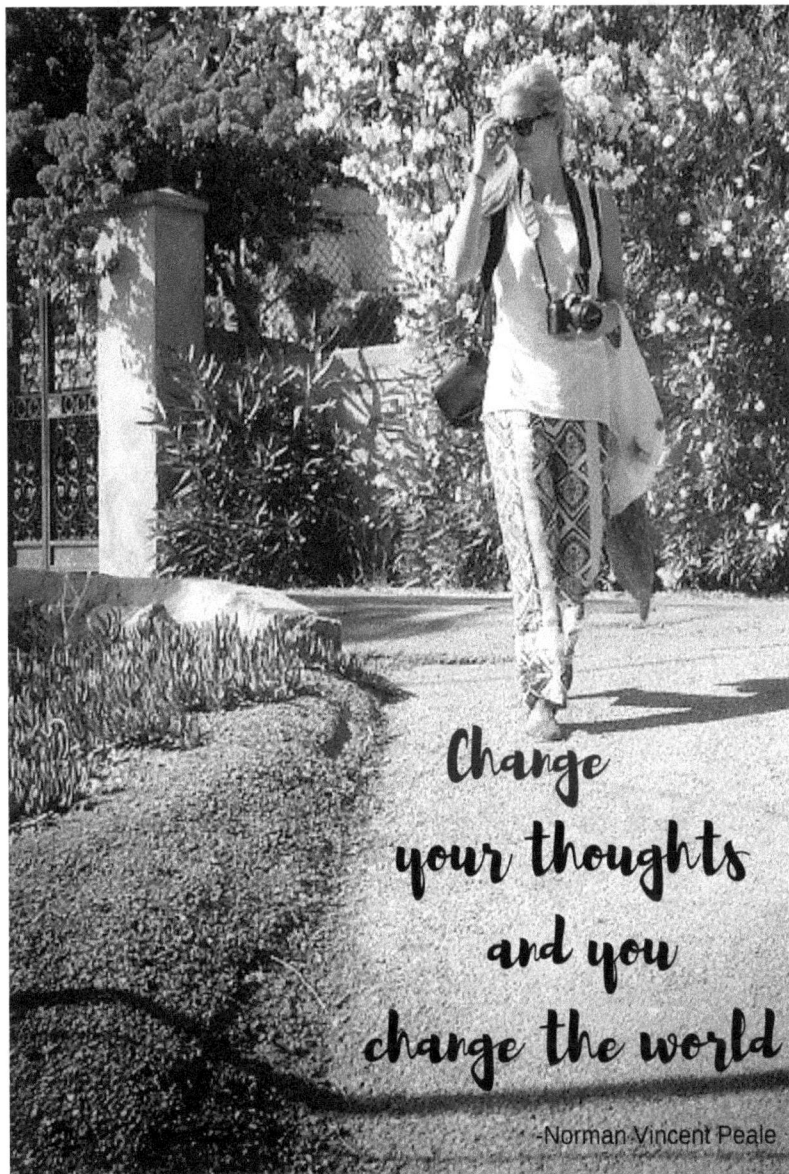

Change
your thoughts
and you
change the world

-Norman Vincent Peale

Part ONE

Nourish

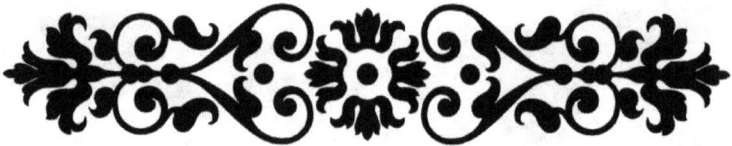

Chapter One

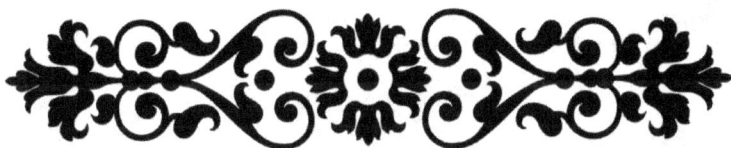

Hydrate

🌿 Drink plenty of pure water

One of the most important things you can do for your health is to ensure you are well-hydrated with plenty of high-quality water.

Our bodies are made up of 60-70% water.[vii] It is the main delivery system for nutrients to your cells, and is required for the removal of toxins. If you aren't getting enough water, the toxins can't be flushed out, and will damage your body.

Water lubricates your joints, and aids in most of the billions of processes going on in your body at any time. We need water for our bodies to function properly. You can go without food for weeks, but you can only survive without water for days.

The reality is that most people don't drink enough water.

Symptoms of dehydration can be vague, and therefore easily ignored.

Do you suffer from any of these?

- Thirst
- Constipation
- Heartburn
- Dry, flaky, wrinkled skin, with a lack of 'bounce'
- High blood pressure
- Headaches
- Fatigue
- Dry, chapped lips[viii]

Everybody has a different water requirement. Although many health professionals recommend 6 - 8 x 250ml glasses a day of water, you may need more, or even less, depending on your size and activity, and medical conditions.

When you become thirsty, your body is telling you to drink, and has lost 1-2% of its total water. It is a sensitive gauge of your body's hydration, and as long as you listen to it, you are unlikely to become seriously dehydrated. It is a myth that you are already badly dehydrated by the time you feel thirst, unless you have a problem with this function, or have learned not to listen to it. Older people, for example, can lose their sense of thirst, and need to drink several glasses of water a day just to make sure.

Sometimes, thirst can be misread as hunger. So, have a glass of water whenever you first notice you are hungry or thirsty. If you're still hungry a few minutes later, maybe you need food after all!

Your urine is a great indicator of your hydration, and should be a very pale and light coloured yellow. This is a good sign that you are flushing plenty of water through your body. If you are taking vitamins, specifically B2 (Riboflavin), your urine can be a bright, fluorescent yellow. With practice, you can determine from the clarity of your urine if you are well hydrated.

If your urine is a deep, dark yellow, or if you aren't urinating very much, or often, it is likely that you're NOT drinking enough water.

One of the most important things you can do for yourself is to stop drinking soft drinks, fruit juices, sports drinks, and the attractively packaged 'healthy' flavoured vitamin waters. They are full of sugar, or artificial sweeteners, and many different toxins as well.

Clever marketing ploys like pretty, or flashy labels are seductive. They were designed to seduce you to buy. Take the time to read the ingredients and you will be shocked by the chemicals your drinks are spiked with. They are also addictive, and can be surprisingly difficult to quit. If you want a real energy drink, try coconut water, juice or a green smoothie!

A Soda Stream to carbonate your filtered water at home can be a safe, satisfying alternative. Especially for those going through withdrawal from the bubbly sensation of soft drink. You can add freshly squeezed lemon or lime or a drop of food-grade essential oil for flavour to make a delicious drink.

Bottled water is not necessarily a safe option, with many varieties containing contaminants, and not necessarily safer than tap water. There is the added complication of the plastic bottle, both for the environment's sake and for the chemicals that leach out of the plastic, and into the water you are drinking. These wreak havoc on your body by disrupting your endocrine system.

Water quality varies worldwide, and in some cases, bottled water is the best, or only option. Seek reliable local advice.

Healthy Tip

So, how much water do you need? SIMPLE!
Here's the formula:

Body weight in Kgs. = Litres of water required
    30   per day, up to max 4 L.

For example: For a 70 kilogram person:

$$\frac{70}{30} = 2.3 \text{ litres per day}$$

Filter your water

If possible, even the water you bathe and shower in should be filtered. While tap water in Australia is relatively safe, it contains many added chemicals, plus those that have found their own way into our water supply.

Chlorine, or the alternative *chloramine*, is only one of the many chemicals found in our 'safe' water supply. It is only there in low doses, enough to kill pathogens such as Cholera, Typhoid, E. coli, and Giardia, but it also kills the 'good' bacteria in your gut.

Fluoride is another additive, intended to ensure we have healthy, strong teeth. There is an ongoing debate about this chemical though, as it has also been shown to cause problems such as fluorosis of the teeth, bone loss and a myriad of other health concerns - from Attention-Deficit Hyperactivity Disorder, lethargy and gastrointestinal problems, to thyroid disease and increased cancer rates.[ixx][xi]

Many other chemicals can be found in our tap water too, including fertilisers, pesticides and heavy metals.

The two main water filters that can be used to filter your tap water are Carbon filters and Reverse Osmosis filters, and these come in many different types and sizes.

Carbon filters are the most common filters and can be positioned on the kitchen bench, or under the sink, and are relatively inexpensive. The cartridges require changing at least annually, for them to work well. These do a good job of removing heavy metals and chlorine, but they don't remove fluoride.

There is a whole house carbon filter system available, which is great as all the water entering the house is filtered, thereby also reducing the toxins in your shower and bath.

Alternatively, as a less expensive option, and in addition to a kitchen sink system, a shower filter can be fitted easily and cheaply to protect your absorbent skin and lungs from taking in the toxic chemicals in your shower water. Absorbing chemicals through skin and lungs can be worse than drinking them in, as the toxins have a more direct and instantaneous route into your blood stream.

Reverse osmosis filters are another alternative, and do a better job of removing chemicals, including fluoride. They are more expensive however, and have the additional effect of removing the beneficial minerals and denaturing the water. This water then needs to be restored by adding minerals through a final filter, to make it whole again.

If you are on a strict budget, at least buy a carbon filter each for your kitchen tap and shower. If you can afford it, buy a whole house filter, and a reverse osmosis filter for the kitchen sink (this requires a separate tap) to remove the fluoride from your drinking and cooking water.

Healthy Tip

Drink the juice of 1/2 a lemon in 600 ml of
pure water every morning on rising to:

- Improve your digestion
- Flush out your liver & lymphatic system
- Boost your Vitamin C intake
- Help maintain a healthy weight

Action Plan

1. Drink plenty of pure water!
2. Stop drinking soft drinks (even diet drinks), sports drinks and flavoured waters. Replace them with clean, pure water.
3. Filter your water.
4. To help you give up the soft drinks, and add variety, try raw vegetable juices, fresh coconut water, and a soda stream.

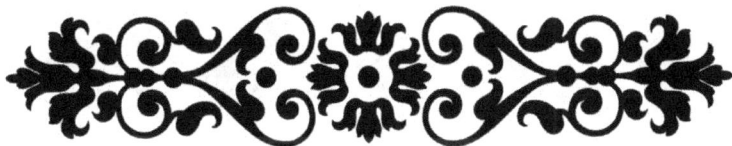

Chapter Two

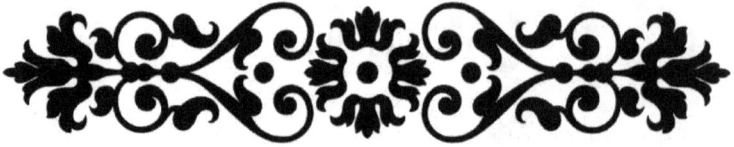

Eat To Nourish Your Body And Mind

"The food you eat can be either the safest and most powerful form of medicine or the slowest form of poison."

— Ann Wigmore

Making simple changes to the food you eat will radically improve how you look and feel in a very short amount of time.

Your body is constantly replacing its cells using the nutrients and chemicals from the things that you ate, drank and absorbed over the last few months - which are coursing through your bloodstream.

Imagine the difference in the quality of the cells that are made from a healthy clean-eating, well-hydrated lifestyle, as opposed to one where fast food and chemicals are regular contributors.

🌿 **A whole food, nutrient-dense diet is a powerful tool for getting yourself feeling on top of the world.**

Processed foods are high in sugar, fructose, refined carbohydrates and artificial ingredients. More than half of the calories in the average diet these days come from flour, sugar and industrial seed oils. They are addictive and satiate your immediate hunger but contain very little in the way of nutrients, fibre and water. It is these 'empty calories' in our processed foods diet (think white bread, burgers, pizza and chips, and the pre-packaged foods in the supermarket aisles) that are currently causing the epidemic of heart disease, fatigue, diabetes and obesity. They are designed to make you overeat, and encourage cravings for more.

These same processed foods trigger chronic inflammation in the body, which is the root of the modern disease epidemic - from cardiovascular and autoimmune diseases, to allergies and arthritis.

The nutrients, fibre and water, found in real whole foods make our bodies feel satisfied, and tell us it is time to stop eating. Swapping processed foods for real food may be the only solution needed to improve your health and get you back to your optimal weight.

A healthy approach is a combination of the principles behind the "Paleo" and "Weston A. Price" methods of eating. They include nourishing, healing, and traditional foods that have always been the mainstay of the human diet before boxes, plastic bags, refined grains and processing came along.

It's simple: eat plenty of fresh vegetables, some good quality meats, healthy fats, some nuts and fruits, pure water and other healthy drinks, and some superfoods for extra nutrients.

Superfoods are foods that are known to be nutritionally dense and therefore especially good for your health.

Processed food is any food that is pre-packaged and has multiple ingredients - and should be avoided. Once you get off the fast, fried, sugar and flavour-enhanced foods, you will really enjoy the abundant flavours and textures of real food and the health benefits that come along with this way of eating. And remember, food is meant to be enjoyed!

🌿 Aim for three to six meals a day

It's good to allow your digestive system to rest between meals, and eating frequently will simply interrupt that rest. If you are eating real, nutrient-dense meals with plenty of quality fats, three meals a day will be enough to keep you energetic and feeling satisfied. Snacks might even become a thing of the past!

🌿 Avoid excessive carbohydrates and sugar

When you eat sugar and other simple carbohydrates, they are broken down and digested very quickly, and rush straight into your bloodstream. This often causes a rush of energy. Your body then responds to this sudden spike in blood sugar by releasing insulin to remove the excess from your blood. The blood sugar lowers as a result of the insulin doing its job, resulting in a desire for more quick-release simple carbohydrates, and so the sugar-craving cycle continues.

If you have been consuming mainly simple carbohydrates for a long time, your body can develop a resistance to insulin and leptin (which is responsible for turning on and off hunger), requiring it to produce more and more of these hormones to do their job. The body then loses touch with its own signals to stop eating or burn body fat. Even eating small amounts of grains and fruits can be a problem for some people. Your body forgets how to burn its stored fat because it is easier to burn the ever available supply of glycogen, the product of the simple carbohydrates.

The result is constant hunger and sugar cravings and the storage of body fat, particularly around your tummy.

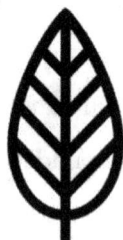

Healthy Tip

Weaning yourself off sugar is one of the most
rewarding actions you can take.
The sooner you change your eating habits, the
sooner you will be rewarded with improved
energy, normalised weight, better moods and
improved overall health.
Once you have made the shift to avoiding
sugar and reducing carbohydrates from grains,
your cravings for junk food will disappear.

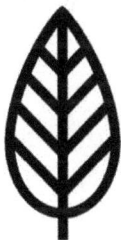

🌿 Eat mostly vegetables

Make vegetables the foundation of your diet.

For optimum health or to heal disorders such as poor sleep, bloating, weight gain, constipation, fatigue, allergies, and a stressed immune system, and to help your body repair from almost every major disease, from diabetes to heart disease and cancer, you need to optimise your diet to improve your insulin and leptin sensitivity.

Insulin and leptin are hormones that work in tandem to regulate energy intake and expenditure. They tell your body whether to burn or store fat.

The best way to improve your diet is by eating mainly vegetables, and crowding out all the less healthy food options. Eat as many non-starchy vegetables as possible, preferably raw, to increase fibre and vital phytonutrients. This way you can overpower the effects of processed, salted, and sugar-laden unhealthy foods.

Try to eat at least 50% of your vegetables raw. Light steaming is another great way to cook your vegetables to retain their nutrients.

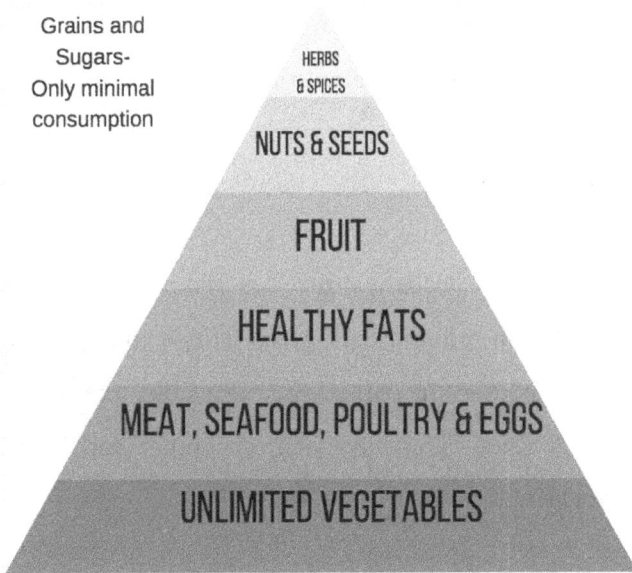

Grains and
Sugars-
Only minimal
consumption

HERBS
& SPICES

NUTS & SEEDS

FRUIT

HEALTHY FATS

MEAT, SEAFOOD, POULTRY & EGGS

UNLIMITED VEGETABLES

The Healthy Food Triangle

Don't worry about overdoing the vegetables. It's hard to eat too many because of their high fibre content.

Malnutrition from a highly processed diet, can lead to overeating. If you are constantly hungry, it may be because you haven't been getting enough nutrients for your body to thrive.

Choose preferably non-starchy vegetables, as the high starch vegetables, such as potato, pumpkin, and corn, convert to glucose when you eat them, triggering your body to release insulin just as if you had eaten something sugary.

While all vegetables are awesome, not all are created equal.

For example, iceberg lettuce has minimal nutritional value compared with red and dark green lettuce and spinach. As a rule, the greener or darker the vegetable, the higher the nutritional value. Think spinach, cucumber and dark green leafy veggies.

Consider juicing as another great way to make sure you are getting more nutrients from vegetables (see page 44).

At first, drinking juice from vegetables may not be very enjoyable. It is an acquired taste. But once you feel the benefits of eating a low carbohydrate and low sugar diet, you will never want to go back!

Healthy Tip

Stock your vegetable drawer
with the best and freshest produce
you can find.
Cutting the fruit and vegetables
into small, ready to eat portions
makes it so easy for snacks
or to take with you on the run!

Protein

Think of protein as the building blocks of the body.

The healthiest proteins come from humanely raised animals. Those who are in their natural environment, on their natural diet, and out in the sunshine. The animals concentrate the nutritional value of the vitamins and minerals they ingest, and pass them onto you.

A vegetarian diet lacks vitamin B12, and many other essential vitamins and minerals. So, take extra care if you choose this course, and be sure to take an appropriate supplement and eat wisely.

❦ Carbohydrates

Your body needs some carbohydrates to function properly. Eat the delicious and nutritious carbs that are good for you – choose mainly vegetables and fruits.

Avoid processed and simple carbs, such as white bread or pasta, and select complex whole grain carbohydrates found in quinoa, sweet potato, and basmati rice instead. They deliver energy more steadily and over a longer period of time, and have a higher nutrient density.

You need to manage the carbohydrates in your diet because they break down quickly into sugar. This sugar is released into the bloodstream, and stimulates insulin. One of the biggest problems in our diets today is the consumption of too much sugar without enough nutrients.

An athlete may need well over 200 grams of carbohydrate a day to perform well. But if you spend most of the day sitting, and not as active, you can thrive on as few as 50 – 100 grams per day. Start with 100 grams and adjust this amount to suit your body.

It's easy to get enough carbs by just eating vegetables, even without grains (such as are used in bread and pasta). You need to experiment with your diet and find what's right for you.

Incidentally, vegetables are also able to provide all of the fibre we need, along with nutrients like folate, Vitamin C, carotenoids, and many other vitamins and minerals.

Fats

We are re-learning the fact that we need to eat fat to be healthy.

Eating a diet high in fats - especially good quality fats from animals and fish, coconut, olives and avocados - will not only make you healthier, but will in fact help you lose weight!

Eat Fat to Burn Fat

Surprisingly, the best way to teach your body to start burning fat is to eat more healthy fats! Minimising carbohydrates and replacing them with healthy fats is the secret to lasting weight loss.

Good fats are essential for optimal health. The membranes of every cell in your body are made of fat molecules. Fats are the perfect energy source, and are required for the absorption of the fat-soluble Vitamins A, D, E and K, which are essential for a healthy immune system amid many other things.

No wonder deficiency in these vitamins is endemic these days, after the past decades of low-fat diets.

Dietary fats are also necessary for the synthesis of normal, healthy cholesterol, which is a building block of steroidal hormones (such as cortisol, oestrogen and testosterone).

Don't be afraid of healthy fats!

Healthy fats include plant fats like coconuts, coconut oil, olives and olive oil, sesame oil, raw nuts (particularly macadamias and pecans) and avocado.

Healthy animal fats and cholesterol rich foods include egg yolks, properly cultured butter from grass-fed cows, as well as their meat.

Always choose food that is closer to its natural form, and remember to maintain healthy portion sizes. If you need to lose weight just adjust your portions!

Cooking with fats

If you are cooking with fats, choose those with a high smoke point, above 180 degrees Celsius (or 350 degrees Fahrenheit), as those that burn and create smoke at low temperatures are shown to damage the cells in your body and cause disease.

Fats that are safe to use when cooking are: ghee, coconut oil, avocado oil, duck fat and lard.

Avoid butter and olive oil for high heat cooking.

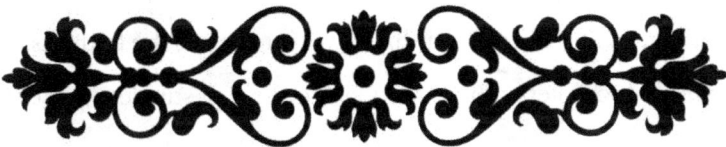

Look for real, nutrient–dense foods, close to their natural state, and buy organic where possible - **whole, unrefined, unprocessed and unmodified.**

Buy your food as if you are hunting and gathering - purchase traditional foods that have always been food.

Eat "superfoods" such as fermented vegetables and drinks, and make homemade bone broth to be used as a drink or to be added to your cooking. (Bone broth is easily made in a slow cooker, which is a fantastic purchase for busy people and worth every cent!)

If you're on a tight budget and can't buy exclusively organic produce, use the Dirty Dozen (plus) and Clean Fifteen lists that are published by the U.S. Environmental Working Group. There doesn't seem to be an Australian version, but U.S. and Australian farming practices are said to be similar.

You can find the lists on the following page. These lists show the fruits and vegetables that are lowest in, or most contaminated with pesticide residues, that are especially toxic to the nervous system. In this way, you can get the benefits of a whole food diet without risking excessive pesticide exposure.

Dirty Dozen

These fruits and vegetables have the highest pesticide residues. Buy organic if possible.

1. Strawberries
2. Apples
3. Nectarines
4. Peaches
5. Celery
6. Grapes
7. Cherries
8. Spinach
9. Tomatoes
10. Capsicum
11. Cherry Tomatoes
12. Cucumbers
+ Kale and Chilli

Clean Fifteen

These fruits and vegetables have the least pesticide residue and may be bought non-organic if necessary.

1. Avocadoes
2. Corn
3. Pineapples
4. Cabbage
5. Sweet Peas
6. Onions
7. Asparagus
8. Mangoes
9. Papaya
10. Kiwi Fruit
11. Eggplant
12. Honeydew
13. Grapefruit
14. Rockmelon
15. Cauliflower

Source: Environmental Working Group, 2016

When you get used to eating this way, it becomes very easy and satisfying in so many ways. You will not want to go back.

Healthy Tip

Eating is an excellent time to practise some mindfulness. This simply means being present in the moment, aware of your surroundings, and what you are doing and thinking.
Simply sitting silently, giving thanks for your food, blessing it and the people you are with, can settle the mind and body and prepare your digestion and greatly improve enjoyment of your meal.

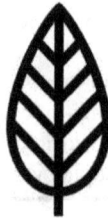

❧ FOODS TO BUY

Buy Superfoods - Nature's multivitamin packed, nutrient–dense foods to keep our bodies healthy and strong.

Meat - look for grass-fed beef and lamb, pastured Australian pork, and non-caged or barn-raised poultry. If this is not possible, do the best you can, and at least try to buy meat from animals that have not been caged and fed antibiotics. Eat organ meats if you are brave enough, as these are jam-packed with nutrients!

Seafood - look for fresh, wild caught fish. If they're not available, buy tinned, wild salmon, sardines, mackerel, or herrings. They're cheaper, more convenient – and rich in Omega 3 fatty acids. The good fats.

Eggs - Try to buy organic eggs from free range chickens. Purchase the freshest you can find as the nutrients gradually dissipate as they age.

Dairy – If you choose to consume dairy foods, the only products I recommend are raw (non-pasteurised) and non-homogenised, which are currently considered illegal in

Australia (unless you have your own cow). This is a source of much ongoing debate. Otherwise, it is best to avoid dairy foods altogether, especially if you don't feel well on them. Dairy foods aren't necessary for calcium, which can be obtained from broth and vegetables.

Vegetables - Buy a variety, and especially dark green leafy vegetables (think spinach, kale, broccoli), avocado (actually a fruit!), asparagus, cauliflower, cucumber, fennel, parsley, tomatoes, turnips, zucchini. Buy fresh and local organic if possible. Before using vegetables, rinse them in a sink full of water with ½ to 1 cup of distilled vinegar for 30 minutes. This will help remove some of the pesticides and herbicides that have been used to grow them if they were not organically farmed.

Nuts - Eat a handful a day of a variety of nuts. Choose more macadamias and hazelnuts and less almonds and brazil nuts to minimise Omega-6.

Olive Oil - Source the most local and cold pressed olive oil in a dark bottle. Buy olive oil from a grower you trust, and check the label for an Australian grown product.

Coconut Oil - Buy raw, organic, extra virgin coconut oil.

Fermented Foods - Sauerkraut, kombucha and kefir. Make them yourself! They are inexpensive and delicious!

Grains - Eat only suitably prepared beans, rice, oats, and some good quality organic sourdough spelt or rye bread if well-tolerated.

Possible occasional sweet exceptions: Dates, raw honey, blackstrap molasses, green (unprocessed) stevia.

WHERE TO SOURCE YOUR HEALTHY FOODS

Search out your local farmers market.

Going to the market every week to get your fresh meat and vegetables is a great social occasion, as well as the perfect place to buy your week's food supply.

Fruits and vegetables from local farms are usually picked within a few days of arrival at the market. They are fresher and will therefore have higher nutrient content. Studies show that spinach loses half of its folate and carotene within a week of being picked. Fruit and vegetables in the supermarket are more likely to have been stored for extended periods of time and sprayed with chemicals to extend shelf life.

Shopping weekly at your local farmers market can help you to plan your meals. It's also very satisfying when you are able to reduce the packaging coming into and out of your home, and only rarely need to visit the supermarket.

🌿 Foods to Avoid

- Modern processed foods, even ones that are labelled "healthy"
- Low fat, low cholesterol foods
- Pasteurised, homogenised dairy
- Refined sugars
- Refined modern wheat flour breads and pasta products
- Artificial sweeteners
- Processed vegetable oils

🌿 Juicing

Regularly consuming fresh vegetable juice is a great way to help you get more concentrated nutrients from your veggies. It also helps if you don't love eating vegetables.

Juicing using a cold-press extractor will help you absorb more nutrients as it helps to "pre-digest" them. It can be a very convenient way to make sure you get a wide variety of vegetables and fruits.

Although it does require some preparation in cleaning and chopping, you can juice enough for the next 24 hours at once. Make sure that you fill the storage jars to the top, to minimise oxidative damage.

Freshly made juice is perfect for when you need a healthy snack on the go!

It is important to remember that vegetable juice made in this way is not a complete meal. It has very little protein and no fat, and should only be used in addition to complete meals for extra nutrients.

Juice also doesn't provide enough beneficial fibre, which is important for your gut bacteria. The fibre is removed during the process.

Consume juices with your meal, or as an additional snack.

Healthy Tip

Limit juicing fruit, apples, carrots and beetroot
as they have a high fructose (sugar) content.
Instead, try half a green apple
with low sugar vegetables
like cucumber, celery, leafy greens and some
ginger and lemon.

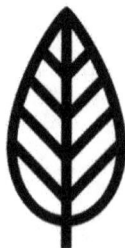

GREEN JUICE RECIPE

Supercharged, detoxifying and anti-inflammatory.

Ingredients:

- 4 stalks celery
- 1 cucumber
- ½ green apple (or beetroot, or carrot)
- handful spinach, kale or substitute green leaves
- ½ inch piece fresh ginger and/or turmeric
- ½ cup coconut water

Push the greens through a juice extractor first, followed by the other ingredients, and into a small jug. Stir in coconut water. Pour into serving glasses.

Smoothies

Smoothies are another way to enjoy a nutritious selection of fruit, veggies and superfoods.

A green smoothie is a whole food, complete with fibre and nutrients, and is quicker to make if you're on the run.

You can add soft ingredients like avocado, nut butters, goji berries and protein boosting powders and superfoods. Get creative! Throw all your favourite healthful foods in a high speed blender and blend until smooth.

Drink slowly to make sure your digestive system has time to do its' work properly.

GREEN SMOOTHIE RECIPE

Ingredients:

- 1½ cups baby spinach leaves
- ½ small banana
- ½ green apple, peeled, cored and chopped
- ½ small lebanese cucumber
- ¼ ripe avocado
- ½ cup coconut water

Blend all ingredients together. Serve in a glass and enjoy! Best served cold.

If you don't have a great blender, blend the spinach leaves and coconut water together first, and then add the other ingredients to ensure it's smooth!

🌿 Fermenting

Eating fermented foods is one of the best strategies to increase beneficial gut bacteria, and promote digestion and immunity. Yoghurt, kefir, kombucha and sauerkraut are great sources of natural, healthy bacteria.

Choose yoghurt that is made from the best quality, full-fat whole milk you can find, without added sugar or pectin, or any thickening agents (the last two are an indication that the bacterial count in the yoghurt will not be high).

Fermented foods are delicious! They can be made easily at home and will provide nearly the same number of good bacteria as an expensive bottle of probiotic supplements at a fraction of the cost.

Healthy Tip

Fermented foods are Superfood Number One!
Add kefir to smoothies for a
refreshing probiotic boost.
Consume sauerkraut as a condiment.
Start slowly with half a teaspoon and
work up to a few tablespoons a day.

🍃 Soaking

Nuts, seeds, grains and legumes contain phytates that reduce the bioavailability of some of the nutrients. They should be soaked before eating to make them easier to digest and to maximise the bioavailability of the nutrients they contain.

Soak nuts overnight and dehydrate them with a food dehydrator, or in an oven on 65 degrees celsius - for 12 to 24 hours. Dehydrated nuts are crunchy and delicious!

Some nuts like raw macadamia nuts and cashews don't require soaking.

🍃 Sprouting

Sprouts are among the most nutrient-packed foods you can eat, and are easy and inexpensive to grow at home. Adding sprouts to your diet will supercharge your nutrient intake!

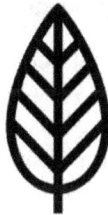

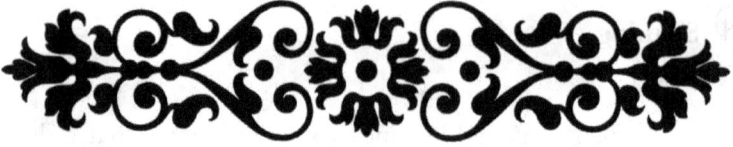

Action Plan

- Find your local farmers markets and buy your food there every week. You are much more likely to get healthy, organic, fresh food with higher nutrient value. It's also likely to be cheaper than you would find in the supermarket!

- Eliminate processed and inflammatory foods such as grains (and in particular those high in gluten) and refined sugar. Start reading the ingredient labels on your food.

- Sit down and eat mindfully. Take ten deep breaths before starting a meal. Rushing will prevent the proper breakdown of protein, and cause bloating and indigestion.

- Avoid drinking while you are eating a meal, because it dilutes the digestive juices. Small sips are okay!

- Add a tablespoon of apple cider vinegar in a glass of water before meals, or add it as a dressing to your salad. Look for one that is unfiltered and still contains the bacterial 'mother'. You should be able to see strands of proteins, enzymes and friendly bacteria.

- Take a probiotic supplement or eat probiotic foods like sauerkraut with meals to help with your digestion.

- Chew slowly, at least 20 times for each mouthful, to break down fibres in your food and mix it with the enzymes in your saliva. This is known as pre-digesting, where carbohydrates begin to be broken down, and is a very important part of the digestive process.

Everyone is different, so listen, learn and experiment, to discover how best to support your body.

If you have extra issues that could be diet-related, it may be best to take a stricter stance and follow an elimination program to pinpoint the foods that are affecting you.

If this all feels overwhelming, seek help from a qualified nutritional therapy practitioner.

Chapter Three

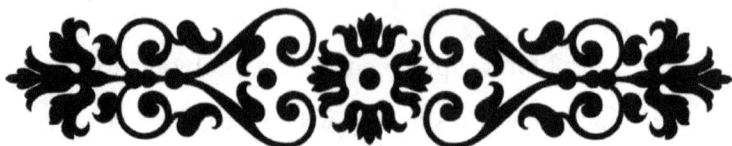

Food For Your Skin

Looking back, I'm surprised at how I used to take my skin for granted, as it quietly goes about its job of protecting my body. It never really occurred to me that everything I put on my skin would be absorbed further than the first layer of skin cells! I thought the skin was a barrier - right? I certainly didn't think of it as a living thing. And I trusted blindly that the manufacturers wouldn't put anything in their products that could harm us. Now I know differently.

Absorption of chemicals through the skin and into the bloodstream depends on the concentration, duration of contact, and solubility of the element. Cosmetics and moisturisers are the perfect delivery system since they are designed with absorption in mind.

Have you ever paused to look at the ingredients on the labels of your favourite skin, hair, nail and dental care products? Heaven knows what some of these unnecessary and sometimes dangerous chemicals are doing to us.

While we're working on the health of our insides, let's have a look at how our inner health is affected by what we put on the outside.

Some of the most common ingredients to avoid include Triclosan, Benzalkonium Chloride, DEA, Diethanolamine and Cocamide DEA, Propylene Glycol, Aluminium, Parabens, Sodium Lauryl Sulfate (SLS), Sodium Laureth Sulfate (SLES) and Phthalates. These toxins increase product shelf life, and add texture or lather, and most are known carcinogens.

On quieter days, I have spent hours in supermarkets and chemist shops scanning the ingredients of products such as toothpaste, shampoo, and body wash that don't contain unnecessary chemical additives.

Toothpaste nearly always contains Triclosan, an antibacterial chemical used in a multitude of household products - known to stay permanently in your body, and Fluoride (there is an ongoing debate about this chemical). Triclosan, for example, has been shown to kill human cells. It acts as an endocrine disruptor and when combined with water, produces chloroform, which is a known carcinogen.

Body wash and shampoos usually contain Sodium Lauryl Sulphate, petroleum by-products, and fragrances - plus other unnecessary chemicals that can damage our bodies.

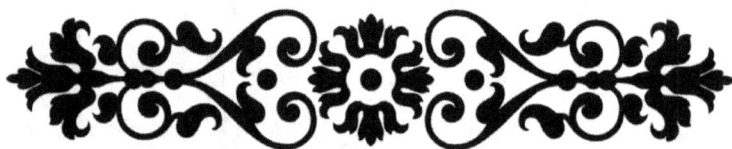

HOW SHOULD WE CARE FOR OUR SKIN?

The face and body care products you use should be as clean and unprocessed as the food that you eat.

Cleansing

Coconut oil and jojoba oil are great for cleansing the face. Just massage them onto your skin and wipe off with a clean, warm face washer.

❦ Toning

Combine one part of good quality, unfiltered apple cider vinegar with five parts of purified water. If the smell is strong, add some essential oils. This toner does a great job of soothing and rebalancing the pH of the skin.

❦ Moisturising

Choose one or more of the following oils below. Place one teaspoon in your palm and using two fingers of the other hand, gently dab over entire face. Then press your palms together and distribute evenly over your neck, chest and shoulders.

- Jojoba Oil (for all skin types, especially for rosacea, acne, eczema)
- Olive Oil (extra-nourishing oil, great for dry skin)
- Avocado Oil (eczema, psoriasis, or sensitive skin)
- Coconut Oil (all skins and also great for fungal infections)
- Macadamia Oil
- Hemp Seed Oil
- Rosehip Seed Oil
- Apricot Kernel Oil

Try these mixed or alone for cleansing and moisturising your face and body. I use them all depending on the time of day and the season, as some feel too heavy for summer. I use hemp seed oil and olive oil in winter when I need extra moisture.

I also add pure essential oils, such as frankincense and geranium, which are known for their anti-inflammatory and anti-wrinkle properties - and smell wonderful.

❧ Deodorant

Bicarbonate soda can be lightly dusted under your arms with a shaving or makeup brush for a great deodorant. If that's too strong, mix it with cornstarch, which can give the added benefit of acting as a mild anti-perspirant. If your skin is sensitive, you can also combine it with some coconut oil. (Apply lightly to make sure your clothes aren't marked.)

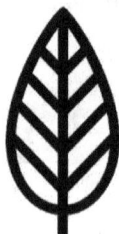

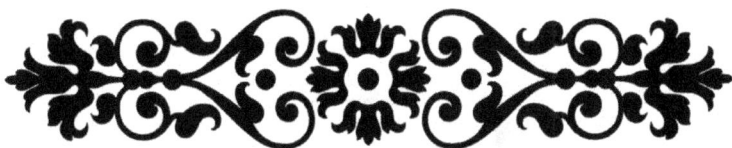

Action Plan

- Look closely at the labels on the cosmetics and other products in your bathroom, and choose to cut back on chemical exposure where you can.

- Keep some bicarbonate soda, apple cider vinegar, coconut oil and pure essential oils on hand in the bathroom, so you can easily make healthier choices.

- Healthy deodorants and skin care products are becoming more readily available and can be found at markets or health food stores. Look for products that only contain very safe ingredients that you recognise: like coconut oil, arrowroot, beeswax and shea butter.

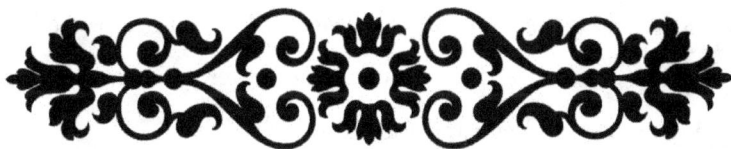

Chapter Four

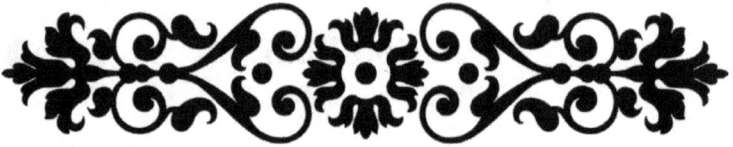

Green Cleaning

While we are avoiding toxic chemicals in the food we eat, the water we drink, and the products we use on our skin, we also need to consider reducing the toxins in our environment.

Our modern homes are often full of furniture, carpets, paints and plastics which emit fumes we are not aware of. Firefighters are aware of this phenomenon, because a fire that took 15 - 20 minutes to engulf a house 30 years ago, now takes only 2 or 3 minutes. This is due to the newer petroleum-based products used in beds and furniture.

Chemicals are absorbed through our skin from contact,

and into and through our lungs from breathing toxic fumes. It's only a matter of seconds before they are circulating in our bloodstream.

These chemicals can stay permanently in your fat and other body tissues.

While moving house or removing furniture may not be an option for you, take care to thoroughly ventilate your home daily with fresh air.

Utilise green cleaning to cut down your exposure to toxins as much as possible. By using fewer chemicals that are known to cause asthma, eczema, allergies, and other autoimmune diseases, you may find some of your ailments mysteriously disappearing.

Our grandparents' generation did not have this toxic load of unnecessary chemicals added to everything in their world.

I know that until recent years, I hadn't stopped to think too much about it. Cleaning products were all about convenience. I was hypnotised by years of heavy advertising by the chemical companies.

A single spray may not cause too much obvious harm, but toxic chemicals are known to build up in our environments and are particularly evident in carpet dust and in the air we breathe.

Making your own cleaning products is cheap, easy and much healthier for you, your family and the environment.

There are so many toxic chemicals out there to avoid - going back to absolute basics can be the safest way to go.

🍃 Microfibre Cloths

Having spent my life nursing and being a mum, I've done a lot of cleaning in my time.

The recent innovation that has made my life so much easier is the microfibre cloth. They are cheap and easy to buy, and a must for chemical-free cleaning. More hygienic than normal fabrics, they can be used to clean without any harsh detergents or chemicals at all.

These cloths aren't advertised heavily because the cleaning industry can make so much more profit from selling industrial strength cleaning chemicals to wage the "war on germs". Our homes don't need these toxic chemicals!

Unlike traditional materials with relatively thick fibres in a flat weave, these cloths work because they have millions of microscopic fibres which grab the dirt and sweep it away, and then keep it trapped until it is washed. They have to be washed separately after use, or they won't lose the dirt, and will just collect more in the wash! Follow the instructions on the pack for optimum care. A bonus is they last forever (almost)!

You will need to experiment when you first start to use microfibres, as you will immediately be inclined to flood them with water and detergent, but they usually only need a little water - and no chemicals!

There are also some great mops made with microfibre, and they are available cheaply in supermarkets. I've been using the same ones for years and prefer them to the heavy old-fashioned bucket-type mop.

HOW TO USE MICROFIBRE

- Dusting
- Washing up cloths in the kitchen
- Wiping down the shower and bath after use
- Cleaning surfaces such as bathroom and kitchen benches
- Cleaning mirrors and glass- dampen a corner to rub away marks and then use the rest of the cloth to shine
- Mopping floors

🌿 Green Cleaning Ingredients

There are times when even microfibre isn't enough, and you need some extra scouring or mould-removing power.

Even in the large public hospitals I work in, only very mild detergent is used in cleaning, unless there's a patient with a 'superbug'. Only then is the immediate environment cleaned with bleach or a strong chemical in a very controlled manner.

Cleaners using harsh chemicals can often suffer after years of exposure. They can find their breathing and skin affected due to long term use.

When I learned about the toxic nature of some of the chemicals in the cleaning products we were using at home, and that we could easily make healthier ones, we started to make our own with some products that are just as comfortable in the food cupboard as in the chemical cleaning product cupboard I used to have! (Except borax, which while considered safe, should still be kept away from children).

These ingredients have been around forever, but our generations have forgotten how to use them because of the convenience of store-bought products and the massive advertising we have been subjected to.

These humble ingredients are eco-friendly, non-toxic, cheap and versatile:

- Bicarbonate soda
- White vinegar
- Citric acid
- Borax (use caution with this, keep out of reach of children and don't ingest, however still considered safe)
- Hydrogen peroxide 3%
- Lemons
- Castile soap
- Washing soda
- Essential oils

Here are some ways to use them as an alternative to toxic and expensive household products.

All-Purpose Cleaner

- Dissolve 4 tbsp. bicarbonate soda in 1 litre of warm water for general cleaning.

- Sprinkle bicarbonate soda on a damp cloth to wipe down kitchen and bathroom surfaces as a cleaner and deodoriser.

- Make a paste from bicarbonate soda and water for a good all-purpose cleaner.

- A stronger all-purpose cleaner can be made with 1 tsp. borax, ½ tsp. washing soda, 1 tsp. liquid castile soap and several drops of essential oils in 2 cups of warm (pre-boiled and cooled) water, and mix in a spray bottle.

- A scouring powder can be made with 1 cup bicarbonate soda, ½ cup salt and ½ cup borax. Put in a shaker. Moisten surface with vinegar for extra power!

- Dunk the cut side of a lemon half in baking soda to clean countertops. Leave for a couple of hours to remove stains, then wipe off.

- Essential oils make a great addition to any cleaning mix as they are generally antibacterial and will also melt away many oil and grease marks.

Glass Cleaner

- 1 part vinegar with 1 part water makes for a perfect smear–free shine especially when buffed with a microfibre cloth.

Toilet Cleaner

- Sprinkle bicarbonate soda in the bowl, squirt with vinegar and scour with a toilet brush to clean and deodorise.
- For extra help with mineral deposits in the bowl, sprinkle citric acid in liberally and leave overnight, you will be amazed at the result!
- Hydrogen peroxide 3% works well as an antibacterial agent, to wipe down toilet and bathroom surfaces if someone at home has been sick.
- A drop or two of essential oil inside the toilet roll or on the microfibre cloth you are using gives a lovely clean scent and has the added benefit of its antibacterial properties.

Drain Cleaner

- Pour bicarbonate soda down the drain, followed by vinegar. Allow the mixture to foam for a few minutes, and then flush with boiling water. Make sure to wear eye protection when using bicarbonate soda and vinegar together, as the reaction can be quite explosive!

Tile and Grout Cleaner

- Moisten 2 cups of bicarbonate soda into a smooth paste and scrub into the grout with a toothbrush and sponge. Rinse thoroughly.
- Hydrogen peroxide 3% can be used in a spray bottle straight, (or try diluted half and half with warm, boiled water). To safely bleach remaining mould stains leave for an hour and wipe down.

Cleaning Refrigerators

- Clean inside and out with 2 tbsp. bicarbonate soda dissolved in 1 litre of warm water, rinse.
- An open pack of bicarbonate soda left in the fridge will absorb musty smells.

Pots and Pans

- For burned-on food, sprinkle on 2 tbsp. bicarbonate soda, splash on some vinegar and watch it fizz off. Alternatively, for a bad pot burn, add some water and gently simmer for a few minutes. Turn off the heat and soak overnight until particles soften and are loosened.

Oven Cleaner

- Spread a paste of bicarbonate soda on gently warmed (<100° Celsius) oven surfaces avoiding elements and leave overnight with a bowl of water to moisten. Wipe over in the morning.

Carpet Cleaning

- Sprinkle bicarbonate soda on carpet before vacuuming as a deodoriser/freshener.
- Stains and grease spots can be removed by rubbing gently with bicarbonate soda, leave overnight to dry and vacuuming thoroughly in the morning.

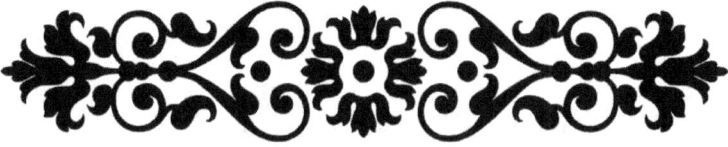

Action Plan

- Are you still using the "Call the poison centre if you ingest, breathe or look at this in the wrong way" type cleaners? Check the ingredients in your cleaning products and replace them with safer healthier options.

- Experiment with natural ingredients singly or combined.

- Take small steps until all your cleaners are natural and/or homemade.

- Buy some microfibre cloths in different colours for different jobs in your workspace and at home.

- Buy some reusable spray bottles to make up with ready for action homemade sprays.

- Purchase some old-fashioned, but hard-working items to experiment with:
    - Bicarbonate soda (Don't worry, it's all naturally aluminium free)
    - White vinegar
    - Citric acid
    - Borax

o   Pure soap flakes or castile soap

o   Hydrogen peroxide 3%

o   Lemons

o   Essential oils

If you prefer the convenience of a store-bought product, there are cleaning products available that have been made with your health in mind. Be sure to read the labels carefully for the ingredients!

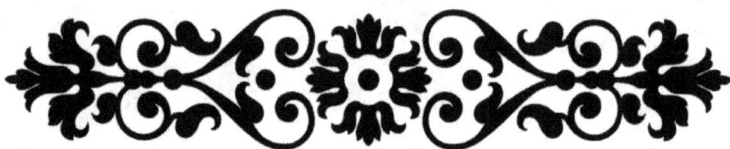

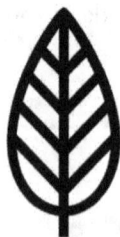

Part TWO

Cherish

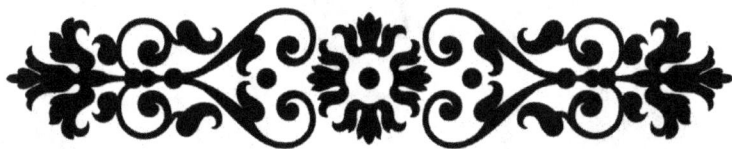

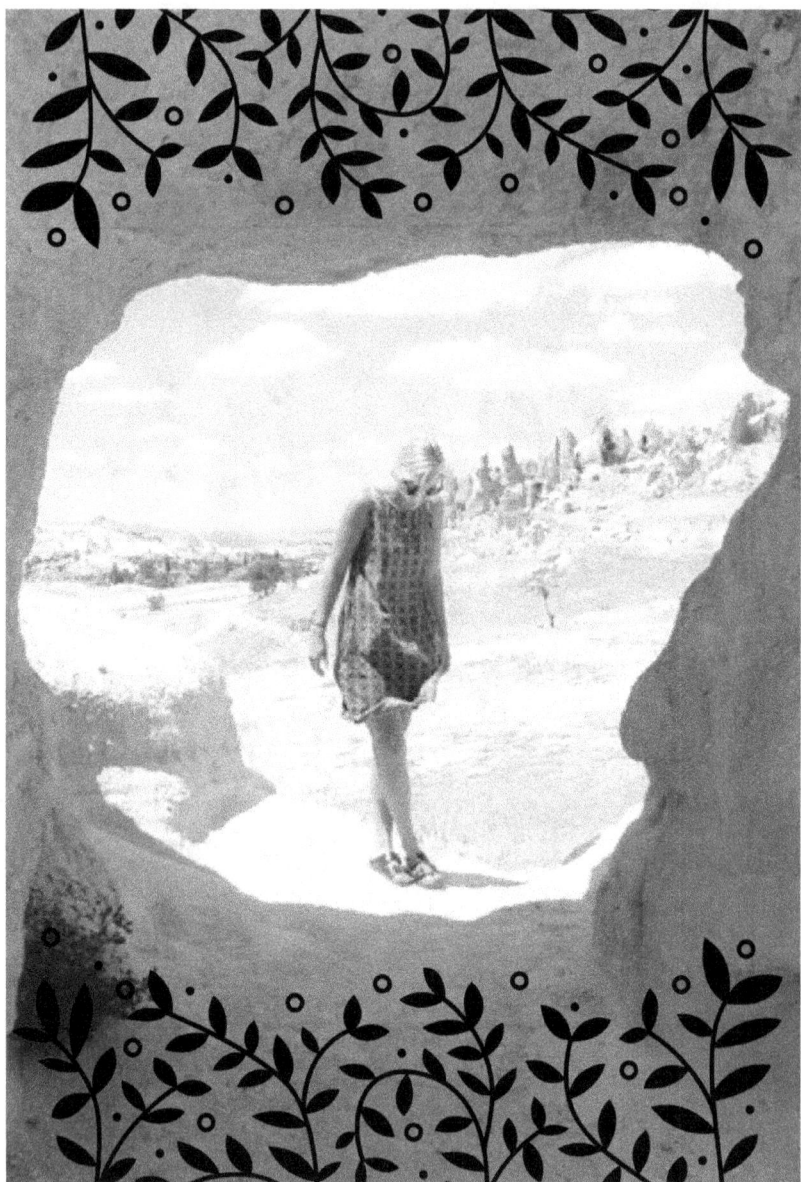

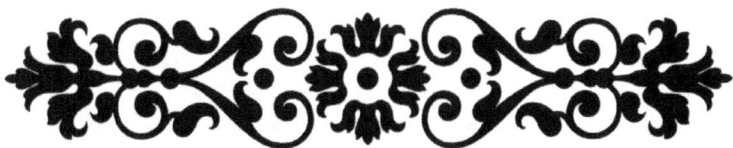

Alex

Over the last decade, Alex had seen countless doctors. She was told her unrelenting exhaustion was just a stage which she would grow out of.

She had almost given up.

As her Health Coach, I encouraged her to have one more try.

We found an Integrative General Practitioner, who ran every blood test under the sun, and shed some light on the way she was feeling.

She discovered imbalances with thyroid hormones, cortisol, MTHFR genetic mutations, pyroluria, and a number of nutrient deficiencies and is treating them naturally where possible.

With ongoing support, she has found that diet and lifestyle factors are just as important as any medication or supplements for healing.

If you are suffering from an autoimmune disorder, fatigue, depression, or any other condition, you need to take a comprehensive approach to healing.

It is important to heal our whole selves: minds, bodies, and the mind/body connection.

Alex is now enjoying life again and living a healthy, happy, vibrant life and maintaining her balance of food, exercise, sleep and fun.

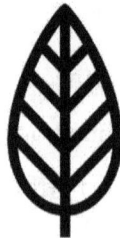

Chapter Five

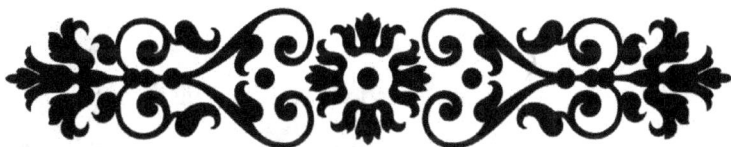

Move

"*Warning: being still is detrimental to your body*"

- Katy Bowman

Modern life and its conveniences have freed up a lot of our time and energy, while mentally, we are left feeling exhausted and overwhelmed by the 24/7 constant connectivity.

It's much harder to be mindful when we are not as active, and our minds work overtime with twenty-four hour a day stimulation. No wonder rates of mental illness have increased along with obesity, diabetes and depression, to name a few!

We've tried hard to exercise more and eat less.

Something isn't working.

Even if you are very fit and work out regularly at the gym, recent studies have shown that sitting for most of your day still increases your risk of premature death.

We are spending hour after hour in our chairs, without moving - and becoming fatter, sicker and more fatigued.

It is now understood that constant movement is essential for wellness of mind and body.

Movement should not be restricted to blocks of exercise.

Biomechanist Katy Bowman's has a great take on movement: "In the same way eating one meal's worth of calories (700) a day doesn't fuel us in the same way a full 2500 calories does, our approach to exercise –an hour a day– is the equivalent to movement-starvation…

It is critical that we read the fine print on the ergonomic prescription label: **WARNING. BEING STILL IS DETRIMENTAL TO YOUR BODY…."**

In her book, "Move Your DNA", Katy explains that when you move, your muscles fire, which causes your blood to be pumped around in that muscle, pulling in the oxygen needed for fuel, and removing cellular waste, which is being constantly created. Our lack of movement is suffocating our cells because it is frequent movement that drives these essential cellular processes.

Exercising heavily the same way with the same muscles (if, for instance, you are a jogger or cyclist), improves the circulation only for the muscles that are in use and can lead to an imbalance in the strength of your body's muscles.

It seems you can eat the perfect diet, sleep well every night and do everything else we have learned - but without the loads on your cells created by constant natural movement, your optimal wellness will remain elusive.

The constant movement that was once a part of our lives has been 'outsourced.' We have become a nation of sitters. Thanks to the way that we live, the average adult sits for 60% of his or her waking hours, and often much more depending on their job.

We weren't designed to sit all day. So much sitting with not much physical activity can have a profound negative effect on human health. It can cause conditions such as heart disease, weakened bones, and damaged blood vessels.

It is believed that our ancestor hunter-gatherers walked an average of 10,000 steps a day, with frequent bursts of intense activity. They squatted and kneeled, and didn't sit continuously for hours at a time.

In the 1800s, 90% of jobs required manual labour, now it is only 2%.

The new Australian Department of Health guideline[xii] recommends that we should aim for 10,000 steps each day, and at least 150 minutes of moderate intensity, or 75 minutes of vigorous activity each week. They also advocate regular muscle-strengthening activities on at least two days a week to maintain mental health, strength, prevent falls, and reduce the risk of Cardiovascular disease and Type 2 Diabetes.

Minimise the amount of time spent in prolonged sitting. Break up long periods of sitting as often as possible. Be active every day of the week if you can.

You can still keep your office job, you just need to

incorporate some regular movements and postural improvements, even if it is just standing up from your seat every 15 minutes through the day.

You can also add some whole body exercise movements into these 15-minute movement breaks to improve your blood flow.

Try to walk 10 minutes in every hour, instead of doing the 10,000 steps all at once.

While intermittent movement and good posture are essential for optimal fitness, you also need to include some formal exercise to help regulate blood glucose, insulin and leptin levels, as well as strengthen your muscles, lungs, heart, joints and bones, brain function, and the prevention of osteoporosis.

Start gently and gradually increase your program to include all of the following modalities.

Seek professional guidance to help you with a plan that will make sure you get maximum benefit from your hard work!

Healthy Tip

A reminder on your phone or fitness band
can remind you to move
(just choose one that doesn't startle you
every time it activates)!

🌿 **Walk.** 10,000 steps a day, broken up throughout the day.

🌿 **Strength training** (also known as weight or resistance training) has been shown to improve osteoporosis, glucose control and cardiovascular health. Aim for 3 sessions a week.

Interval training is known to improve cardiovascular health, and is based on short bursts of intense exercise interspersed with recovery periods at a slower pace. Aim for 2-3 times a week with a rest between sessions.

Stretching exercises like yoga improve circulation, increase the elasticity of the joints and have the added benefit of a calming effect. They are great to do daily if you can.

If you have any heart conditions or medical concerns, or have not been doing much exercise, ensure you get clearance from your health professional before starting any fitness program.

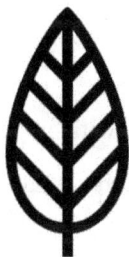

Sophie

Are you feeling exhausted, lacking the motivation to exercise or suffering from recurring injuries?

Sophie had the same experience. After years of spending hours in the gym and hitting the pavement, it came as no surprise that she eventually burnt out.

She made the decision to stop exercising and help her body recover from the thyroid hormone imbalances, adrenal exhaustion and other deficiencies that prevented her from having optimal energy. As her energy improved, she proceeded to walk every day, incorporating yoga and other activities that she enjoys.

She now stays active with yoga, rock climbing, strength training and doing things that make her feel well and happy, without leaving her feeling exhausted and depleted.

Healthy Tip

Walking, yoga and
other low impact activities
help greatly with stress and
get you moving.

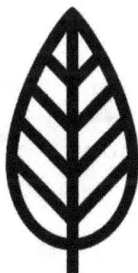

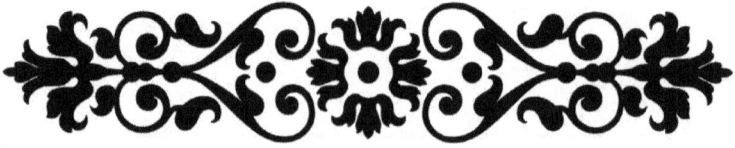

Action Plan

- Just move! Move in different ways. And play.

- Find ways to move that work for you - stand up or sit on the floor, constantly change your seating position to develop strength and alignment throughout the body.

- Discover activities that work for you, not against you!

- Include frequent light activity throughout your day.

- Use the stairs when possible.

- Walk or cycle to work.

- Do your own housework.

- Walk outside barefoot.

- Do your own gardening.

- If you sit, make sure to stand up every 15 minutes.

- Monitor your posture when walking, and sitting in particular.

- Aim for 10,000 steps a day.

- Heal yourself, reduce stress in your life with exercise and enjoyable activities that keep you moving. Have more fun!

- Find a trusted exercise professional to assist you with designing a program to get you safely on track.

- Gradually build up a program of:
  - ✓ Walking 10,000 steps a day
  - ✓ Interval training- intense exercise for several minutes, 2-3 times a week, plus
  - ✓ Strength training 3 times a week, plus
  - ✓ Stretching exercise (like yoga) 3-7 times a week for 10 minutes on waking or at bedtime.

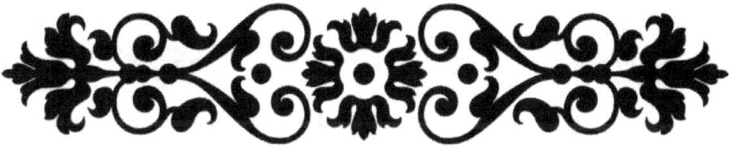

Chapter Six

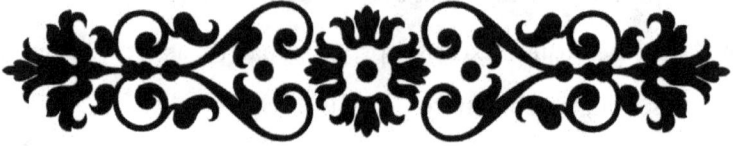

Sleep

"Sleep is the golden chain that ties our health and our bodies together"
- Thomas Dekker c.1600

We've always known sleep is critical to allow your body to repair, regenerate and rebuild. But despite vast amounts of research, we still don't completely understand exactly why we need it. It's still a mystery.

Until relatively recent times, our bodies have run by their circadian rhythms – the twenty-four-hour body clock in the brain. We have evolved to sleep when it's dark and be awake when it's light. It will take many hundreds of generations to adapt to our modern artificial lighting and 24/7 lifestyle.

Melatonin is a hormone that works with the circadian rhythm to induce sleep. In a natural world, free from exposure to artificial lighting from light bulbs and electronic screens, **melatonin levels begin to rise at 7 p.m. and stay elevated until around 7 a.m**. It is first released when the brain discerns that the light is dimming.

Exposing yourself to artificial lighting at night interrupts melatonin production, as does having insufficient light during the day. **Even switching on a bedside light at night is enough to disrupt melatonin production**. Managing your light exposure is crucial to helping maintain normal melatonin levels, and getting optimal sleep.

Recent research[xiii] has found one new and interesting reason for the necessity of sleep - the brain uses sleep to cleanse itself. Brain cells have been found to shrink in size during sleep, allowing the cerebrospinal fluid much greater access to flush toxic waste from the tissues.

One particular waste product identified as being removed in significantly greater quantities during sleep is amyloid–beta, the notorious toxin found in the brains of Alzheimer's sufferers.

Researchers are investigating the hypothesis that if we can improve our sleep, and help clear amyloid-beta from our brains, it is possible to prevent the onset of Alzheimer's disease in some cases. That's a very worthwhile reason to get plenty of good quality sleep.

We spend an average of one-third of our lives sleeping (or trying to). Armed with this information, you should now be more inclined to invest in yourself to establish good sleeping habits.

The Australasian Sleep Health Foundation recommends 7-9 hours of sleep a night for adults to be properly refreshed, and at their best. This varies from person to person. As with all things, every body has different requirements.

Are you suffering from relentless stress and exhaustion? Are you waking up feeling unrefreshed? Are your memory and concentration suffering?

Frequent yawning through the day is a sign that you are not getting enough sleep. If you nod off while sitting or trying to read, you need more sleep.

Poor sleep has also been found to increase your risk of weight gain, weaken your immune response, shorten your lifespan, and accelerate aging.

So you can see why sleep is such a priority for your health and well-being.

❦ ESTABLISH YOUR SLEEP RITUAL

Between a busy social calendar and catching up on TV, facebook and emails, it's easy for sleep to slip from the priority list.

A sleep ritual will help you to achieve the high-quality sleep you need.

- Establish regular times for sleeping and waking. You know best how much sleep you need. What works for someone else might not work for you. We all have different requirements. So base your sleep/wake times according to your body's needs. But remember, the earlier to bed and to sleep the better! The sleep you get before midnight is the most beneficial.

- A warm shower or bath is a great way to wind down and prepare for sleep.

- Epsom salt baths provide a boost in magnesium, which helps create a feeling of relaxation by activating the calming neurotransmitters in the body.

- Add a few drops of soul-soothing essential oils, such as lavender or sandalwood onto your skin or pillow.

- Start preparing for sleep at least half an hour before bedtime.

- Turn down the lights, have a warm bath or shower, read (nothing related to work or study), listen to relaxing music or wind down with your partner or your family.

❧ CREATE A SANCTUARY FOR SLEEP

- Keep your room cool.

- Use blackout curtains where possible.

- Cover any sources of electronic light while sleeping. If you can't remove all sources of light, find a comfortable eye mask.

- Hide your alarm clock so that you can't see the time if you wake during the night.

- Have earplugs on hand to avoid any disruptions during the night (the mouldable soft wax kind are my favourite).

✿ LIMIT EXPOSURE TO ELECTRONICS

- Turn the lights down and light some candles or use a gentle bedside lamp instead. This will assist with the production of melatonin, a naturally occurring hormone that regulates your body's circadian rhythm.

- In the hour before bed avoid using your phone, computer or watching TV. If you must use your phone or computer, try F.lux, a free program that reduces the impact of the light of your screen. If possible, keep all electronic screens outside of the bedroom.

- Find an alternative to using your phone as an alarm, such as an old, unused phone on flight mode, or the old-fashioned variety of clock without any bright screen.

It is believed that electromagnetic radiation (EMR) from wireless internet, mobile phones, cordless phones and your home's power box can reduce the production of melatonin, in turn impacting your circadian rhythm and the quality of your sleep. Turn off your phone, or at the very least, switch it to flight mode.

Healthy Tip

Install a timer on your wireless internet
to turn it off automatically
and mitigate the effects of EMR
while you sleep.

🌿 ESTABLISH A SELF-CARE ROUTINE TO EASE YOUR MIND

It is so important to establish a self-care routine to help you feel relaxed throughout the day and as you prepare for sleep.

Meditation can make you healthier and happier, and more relaxed and ready for sleep. If you have trouble getting into the zone, try a guided meditation.

LifeFlow, Holosync or the more affordable version Insight, are a combination of soul-soothing sounds and vibrational technology (these are my favourite for making meditation so easy when your mind is racing).

🍃 GET OUTDOORS AND CATCH SOME RAYS

Get some sunshine every day, if possible. Let the sun shine on your face, remove your sunglasses (being mindful of excessive sun exposure) and allow natural light into your workspace. Sun exposure during the day strengthens your circadian rhythm and helps melatonin production when the sun goes down.

Fresh air and exercise are also very helpful for achieving quality sleep. Fresh air is often underrated, but it can improve your health and sense of wellbeing.

Avoid moderate to high intensity exercise for 3 hours before bedtime. Exercise produces cortisol, a stress hormone that can affect your sleep.

🌿 EAT RIGHT, SLEEP TIGHT

What you put into your body can make or break your sleep quality. Real food will maintain your blood sugar, insulin and leptin levels, contributing to overall good health and restful sleep.

Although alcohol may help you drift off, it reduces sleep quality and may wake you during the night.

Caffeine is a stimulant, and should be limited to improve your sleep quality. 25% of the caffeine you consume is still in your system 10 hours later! That afternoon cup of tea or coffee may be preventing you from falling asleep at night. You don't have to give up your daily latte, but limit your caffeine intake to the morning hours.

Try foods that promote sleep, such as fish, green leafy vegetables, avocado, walnuts, almonds, cherries, and banana, and drink chamomile tea in the evening.

🌿 WAKING IN THE NIGHT

If you are frequently waking up at night, take note of why so that you can make the necessary changes and avoid it happening again, if possible.

Do you wake up thinking of your to-do list or feeling anxious about life? Stay out of your head! Regular journaling will help you deconstruct your thoughts, process them, and in doing so, reduce your stress.

Do you wake up to go to the bathroom in the night? Limit fluids in the evening to avoid interrupting your sleep.

If you are constantly waking up during the night, and have trouble falling back to sleep, it is important to avoid any unnatural light sources. If you wake up to go to the bathroom, use a torch with an amber light or keep a night light on that won't disrupt your sleep cycle as much as flicking on all the lights. Whatever you do, don't check your phone or any other electronic devices. This will send signals to your body that it's time to wake up.

🍃 STAY OUT OF YOUR HEAD

Keep a gratitude diary or journal beside your bed. This is a powerful tool for being mindful of your blessings, consciously acknowledging your worries, and releasing them to the universe.

If you have trouble falling asleep, or you wake up in the night thinking of all the things you have to do the next day, get organised! Keep a note pad beside your bed and write out a to-do list before bedtime. Then you can sleep soundly knowing that you will remember the things you have to do the next day. Wondering how you will get it all done? Relax. Learn to trust the universe.

If you've tried all these ways of staying out of your head and still can't switch off, keep a meditation track and headphones beside your bed. Even if you can't sleep, you can still relax and allow your brain to rest and restore through meditation.

You can also learn diaphragmatic breathing to slow your heartbeat, and help you drift off to sleep. Armed with this knowledge, you will soon be on your way towards blissful, restorative sleep. We have faith; you can do it!

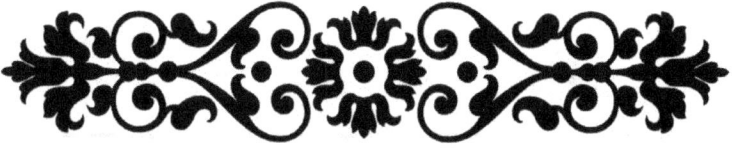

Action Plan

- Expose yourself to bright light during the day.
- Make sleep a priority.
- Establish a relaxing routine to prepare yourself for bed every night.
- Have a relaxing bath or shower before bed.
- Get to bed early enough to get the sleep you need.
- Put a few drops of lavender essential oil on your pillow.
- Leave the electronics out of the bedroom.
- Read a good book to help you relax.
- Use bedside lights with low-blue emission.

Don't add to your stress about sleep by worrying about it! Just maintain a positive attitude, make changes for the better and little by little you will find your sleep improving.

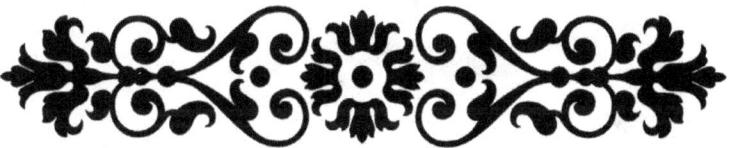

Healthy Tip

When you are healing, listen to your body,
and learn to let go of any feelings of guilt
associated with skipping exercise
in favour of sleep.

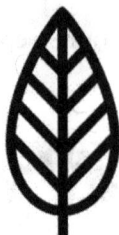

The purpose of our lives is to be happy

Dalai Lama

Chapter Seven

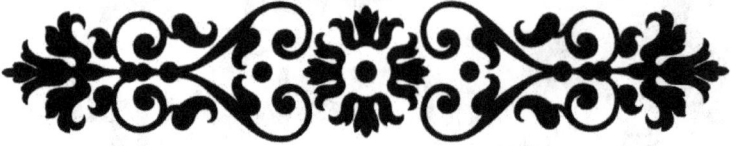

Manage Your Stress

"The purpose of our lives is to be happy"

- Dalai Lama

Stress isn't always bad.

In fact, stress can be a positive thing because it motivates and improves performance, and keeps you focused.

Positive stress is short-term and easy to cope with.

Negative stress feels unpleasant, tends to be chronic, and can lead to mental and physical ill-health.

We are well-equipped for short-term stressful situations where the cortisol and adrenalin, that are designed to help us to survive, disperse quickly once we are out of danger.

Humans have evolved to experience this fight or flight response - and then to continue enjoying life. Finding pleasure and social connection with other human beings acts as an antidote to stress.

In this modern world, we are exposed to constant, chronic, low-grade stress. From the first buzz of the alarm clock, and rushing out the door, to the traffic, work problems, family problems, bills to pay, children to collect and arguments with the neighbours... the list is endless.

Then there are other things that can contribute to chronic stress, such as skipping breakfast, not getting enough sleep, drinking too much coffee, alcohol or energy drinks, even watching a scary movie before bed.

Not getting enough rest between intense workouts can also be a chronic stressor.

Not being able to turn off the turmoil created by thoughts going around and around in your head can be a constant stressor for some.

And then there are the big ones - the death of a family member, divorce, moving house, health problems, losing your job and more. Our bodies aren't designed for chronic modern stress.

The stress response is turned on but never turned off.

You may have noticed how easily you catch a cold when you are in a particularly stressful period in your life.

Chronic stress is a major contributor to immune system disorders.

It also increases your cravings for calorie-dense junk foods, and can lead to leaky gut, inflammation, and susceptibility to infection.

It is such an important piece of the puzzle. If you don't manage your chronic stress well, it can undermine all the other positive changes you are making. **It's just as important to prioritise and build stress reduction techniques into every day, as it is to eat well, and exercise.**

In turn, a good diet and plenty of exercise are priorities for your mental well-being. During exercise, your body increases the levels of endorphins or "feel good" hormones in your brain, while a healthy high-nutrient diet ensures you have plenty of the vitamins available which are known to lower stress hormone levels.

Studies[xiv] have also proven that pleasure and social connection may be as important to our well-being as food, exercise, or sleep.

We also know that the physical connection formed from touching or hugging a friend or family member, cuddling with a pet, even having a therapeutic massage reduces stress-induced cortisol levels. Touch, love, laughter, and fulfilling social interactions increase the hormone oxytocin - which increases feelings of calm and contentment, and reduces anxiety, fear and nervousness. These feelings of social connection are paramount to general health and well-being.

Even a 10 second hug every day can lead to an improvement in your health.

In addition to the power of exercise, diet and physical connection, here are some other ideas that might feel right for you to include in your daily stress management.

🌿 Time Management

It's difficult to stay relaxed and present when you are feeling overwhelmed with commitments. Learning time management skills and establishing boundaries by learning to say no, will go a long way to reducing your stress levels.

🌿 Become aware of your thoughts and change your perspective

Negative thoughts create stress and tension in our bodies. Become aware of your thoughts and change negative thoughts to a more positive outlook.

If you are stressed by circumstances or things you cannot change, try looking at them differently. For example, being stuck in traffic can be stressful, but with a change in perspective it could be a time for catching up on some podcasts or audible books, exercising your pelvic floor muscles, or simply enjoying some solitude.

🍃 Prioritise

Each morning spend some time thinking about what needs to be done that day. Prioritise things that are important and drop the things that aren't. To–do lists are great for this!

Use a large annual wall calendar plus an old-school diary.

Focus on longer term planning, and reach your goals. Get your thoughts and action plans out of your head - and into your diary. If you have a lot happening, it helps to have it all laid out on the wall calendar too.

🍃 Avoid stressed-out individuals

If you are an individual who experiences empathic stress, consider avoiding negative or overly stressed individuals, or even turning off the evening news if it upsets you.

🍃 Learn to accept the things that can't be changed.

Many things in life are not in our control.

🍃 Don't feel that everything has to be perfect.

🍃 **If in conflict with another person, try to get in touch with their feelings and needs.**

> If you can understand where they are coming from, it may be less likely to upset you.

🍃 **Spirituality, meditation and prayer can also be powerful tools for wellness.**

> If any of these resonate with you, take the time to investigate them.

🍃 **Learn to reframe your experiences.**
The weather is not terrible, it is what it is.

🍃 **Be grateful. Say thank you to the Universe daily.**

🍃 **Cultivate empathy and understanding.**

🍃 **Practice acceptance.**

🍃 **Play.**

🍃 **Make sure you have at least a 10-second hug every day, even if you hug yourself!**

🌿 Spend time outdoors exercising.

🌿 Schedule stress management on your calendar to prioritise it.

🌿 Meditate daily, or use yoga or Tai Chi on the days that you are too wound up to relax.

🌿 Scale back your life.

🌿 Make your life more realistic.

🌿 Don't overcommit. Learn to say no.

🌿 Turn off your computer and mobile phone for scheduled periods of time to avoid constant connectivity.

🌿 Laugh. Sing. Spend time with people who value you. The real you.

🌿 Enjoy spending some time alone regularly.

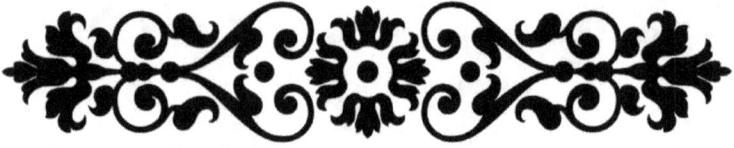

Action Plan

- Reduce the amount of stress you experience by learning to say no, avoiding people who stress you out (when possible), turning off the news, giving up pointless arguments, and addressing physiological problems (such as blood-sugar swings, gut infections, chronic inflammation, and so on) that are taxing your adrenals.

- Reduce the impact of stress you can't avoid by reframing the situation, rethinking your standards, practicing acceptance, cultivating gratitude and empathy, and managing your time.

- Make stress management a priority. Give it as much attention as you give other aspects of staying healthy, such as diet, exercise, and sleep.

- Commit to a regular stress-management practice. Choose a mix of techniques that suit your temperament and lifestyle, such as meditation, yoga, massage, Feldenkrais, mindfulness-based stress reduction, acupuncture, and biofeedback.

- If you're new to stress-management practices, start small and be gentle with yourself. Consider finding a skilled teacher who can help you get started and deepen your practice.

In addition to everything we've listed above, one of the most important things you can do to manage stress is to bring more pleasure, joy, social connection and fun into your life.

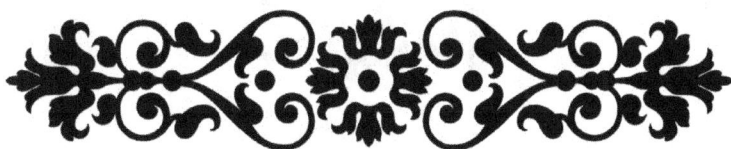

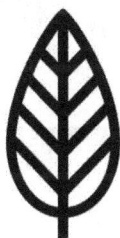

Chapter Eight

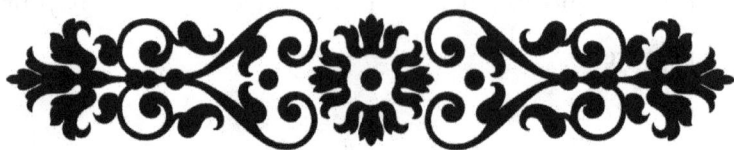

Walk Barefoot

Outside

"If you wish to know the divine, feel the wind on your face and the warm sun on your hand"

- Buddha

On Vitamin D, the grounding effects and the spirituality of nature.

Getting outdoors is beneficial in so many ways. There is more to it than meets the eye.

One of the greatest joys in life is to be able to sit in the sun to absorb the gentle warmth of the sun's rays, or kicking off your shoes and walking barefoot on the earth.

Recent research[xv] indicates it isn't just the good feeling of walking barefoot on the ground that makes the difference. It's about the electrical connection made when your skin makes contact with the ground, and you absorb a steady flow of electrons from the earth.

We are bio-electrical beings, and our every action, movement and thought is powered by electrical energy.

Our bodies are made up of a high percentage of water, in which a variety of electrolytes (charged ions) are dissolved. We are electrical conductors, and the earth is also an electrical body, just like a supercharged battery with an abundant supply of electrons.

Reconnecting to the earth allows these free electrons to help your body neutralise excess free radicals and reduce the inflammation they cause.

Walking barefoot on the grass or along the beach, even swimming in the ocean is therapeutic.

Don't overthink this - just kick off your shoes and walk outside, even if it is just for how good it makes you feel!

🌿 **Sunshine and Vitamin D**

We have all been so thoroughly warned against going out in the sun, with the result that many of us have low vitamin D levels. Sunshine prompts your skin to produce vitamin D, and there are many more benefits that science still doesn't fully understand.

Just as plants require sunlight to grow well, so it is that our bodies need solar energy to thrive.

Vitamin D plays an important role maintaining your health in so many ways, and influences 10% of your genes, making it crucial for your health and well-being.

Your doctor can order a blood test to check your Vitamin D level. Have it checked every 6 - 12 months.

We do need to be careful of the sun and the damage it can cause. However, sensible sun exposure has so many benefits it's worth making the effort to regularly expose your skin safely.

The colour of your skin will tell you when you've had enough sun. Aim to stay out in the sun just long enough to avoid turning pink, with at least 40% of your body exposed.

If you have dark skin, you may require longer periods in sunshine to maintain vitamin D levels in an adequate range.

Always protect your face and eyes by using a good quality sunblock (that protects against UVA and UVB rays) and hat, because the facial skin is usually thinner, more fragile and prone to damage. It also is a relatively small surface area and so doesn't contribute overly to vitamin D production.

Make sure to use sunblock, long-sleeved shirt, pants and hat when you have reached your optimal exposure. Always err on the cautious side - don't allow yourself to get burned as this is when skin damage will occur.

Healthy Tip

Avoid sitting in the sunlight if it is coming through glass.

Sunlight is made up of 95% UVA and 5% UVB rays. The UVA rays are responsible for tanning and damaging skin, and are more able to penetrate materials such as the earth's atmosphere and panels of glass. The UVB rays that produce Vitamin D in the skin are shorter and less energetic and, therefore, less able to penetrate glass.

Remember, if you use sunscreen after you've had your dose of sunshine, choose your product carefully and check for potentially harmful ingredients. Look for one that includes safer ingredients such as zinc oxide or titanium dioxide.

The Spirituality of Being in Nature

There is another aspect to being outdoors that you will intuitively understand - the spirituality of being in nature. The connection with life and the universe beyond our own small world. This is something we often miss in this modern life and it is an underestimated tonic for the soul.

🍃 Walk Barefoot Outside

If you can combine all of these, you'll be living the dream!

Exercise

+ Barefoot Grounding

+ Sunshine

+ Spirituality

= Bliss!

Healthy Tip

Meditation: As you stand, imagine the healing power of the Earth coming up through your bare feet, through every cell of your body and out through the top of your head,and up into the Heavens. Then draw the energy back down through your head and back into the Earth. Breathe deeply and slowly, and enjoy the connection.

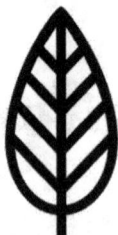

Chapter Nine

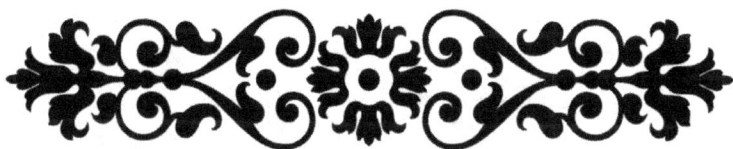

Keep It Going!

🌿 The Recipe for an Awesome Life

Your body is one of Mother Nature's most miraculous accomplishments. **It is a powerful self-healing machine that seeks to stay in perfect health if given the care it needs.**

There is no need to feel overwhelmed by the need for change - any change is worthwhile!

It is easiest to start with small, simple changes and

gradually build your new routines. Choose one or two areas to work on at a time and mark them off as you go.

Write down your health goals in a place you will see them daily.

Make a plan for your week ahead. If you are prepared with food items and expectations, it is much easier to make the necessary changes.

Set simple and achievable goals to help you make lasting positive changes.

Remember that life is a journey, not a destination, and as you follow your path, keep fine-tuning what works best for you. Check in with yourself regularly.

Make sure that any health goals you set are also aligned with your long term happiness.

Start a journal to record your goals and dreams, and set them in concrete. Get into the habit of regularly reviewing your progress.

Recognise your barriers and work on living beyond them.

Remember too that nine out of ten things you worry about never happen.

Enlist your circle of receptive friends, family and co-workers to support you on your journey. Help them understand why you have chosen this path, and they may even join you.

Be aware of, and avoid those who might ambush your efforts, knowingly or unknowingly. There are always people who will undermine your goals, for their own reasons.

It is the people who support you on your path who will help you be accountable, and to reach your goal of extraordinary health, happiness and vitality.

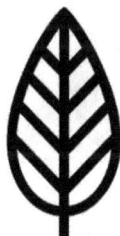

Don't wait until tomorrow to start living - Start now!

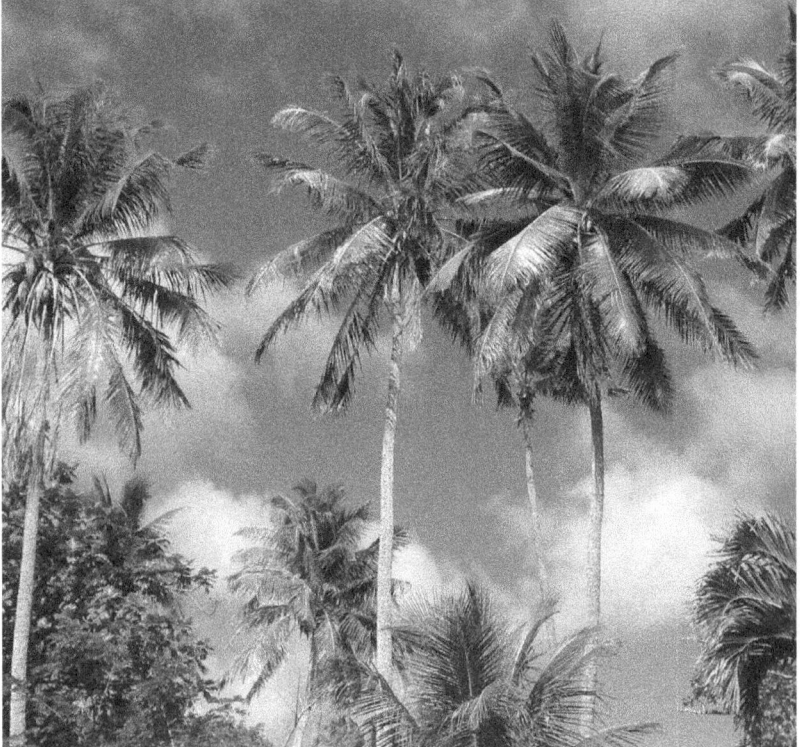

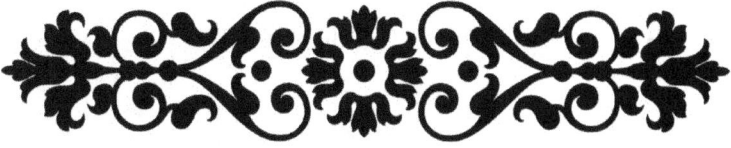

The Great Life Action Plan

🌿 Make an eating plan every week, to prepare ahead. If you are tired and hungry, and there is no food readily available, you are likely to fall back into old habits.

🌿 A weekly trip to the local farmers markets goes a long way towards meal preparation.

🌿 Make sure the food you bring home is organised and ready for the week ahead.

🌿 Cook ahead for the week, if you choose.

🌿 Eat whole foods - real foods.

🌿 Work on eliminating processed foods.

🌿 Add some "superfoods" to your diet every day.

🌿 Hydrate well.

🌿 Drink lemon juice squeezed into filtered water when you wake in the morning half an hour before having anything else.

🌿 Think about how well you digest your food and make improvements with chewing.

🌿 Eat some fermented foods 1 to 3 times a day.

🌿 Be aware of the choices you are making.

🌿 Start reading the ingredients on everything you consume inside and out.

🌿 Avoid chemicals as much as possible in your day to day life.

🌿 Buy some bicarbonate soda to experiment with in cleaning and personal care.

🌿 Remember to take some stress-reducing actions every day.

❦ Find and maintain great, supportive friendships - people who help you be more of who you are.

❦ Find spirituality in something, whether it is yoga, a religion, or a walk in nature.

❦ Walk outside, barefoot, daily, to ground yourself with the earth.

❦ Get sunshine safely 2 or 3 times a week.

❦ Make sleep a priority.

❦ Establish a sustainable exercise program that you enjoy and look forward to.

❦ Start simply, step by step, and build up a lifelong habit of living a vital and beautiful life.

Take note: It may not always be easy. Acknowledge the challenge, and be grateful for where you are on your journey. Making big changes to your diet and lifestyle can be challenging. It may be that you could benefit from the ongoing support of a Health Coach or Nutritionist.

The Ideal Daily Routine

On Rising

- Drink juice ½ lemon squeezed into 600 ml of pure water
- 20 minutes of yoga or journaling

Breakfast

- Yoghurt with berries and a sprinkle of tasty sunflower seeds, or 1 - 2 scrambled eggs with sautéed spinach, mushrooms, and onions.

Lunch

- Large green salad with sprouts, tomatoes, celery, cucumber, dressed with olive oil and balsamic vinegar - and a serving of sauerkraut.

Snacks

- Handful of nuts
- Fresh vegetable juice

Dinner

- Small glass of Kombucha
- Small piece of organic grass fed beef or wild salmon with a variety of steamed vegetables
- 2 - 3 squares of good quality dark chocolate

Make one evening a week electronic free - read a book, have a chat instead.

Hydrate

- Remember to drink plenty of pure water.

Daily activities

Walk 10,000 steps a day, broken up through the day.

Choose 1 of:

- 20 minutes of high intensity interval training or strength training.
- Or 30 - 45 minutes of brisk barefoot walking or gardening.

Include appropriate time in the sunshine.

Evening

- 10 minutes of stretching or yoga before bed.
- 9 - 10 p.m. Prepare for bed.

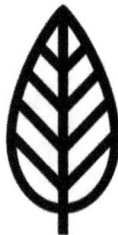

My Perfect Routine

On Rising:

Breakfast:

Lunch:

Snack:

Dinner:

Hydrate:

Daily Activities:

Evening:

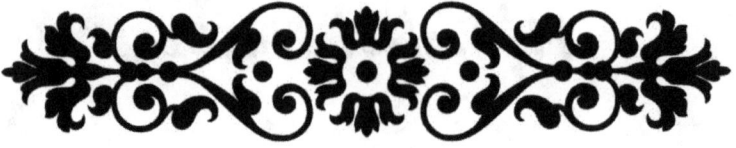

Notes

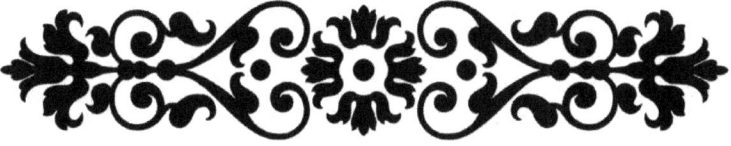

Notes

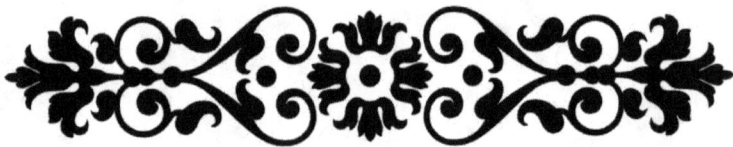

Notes

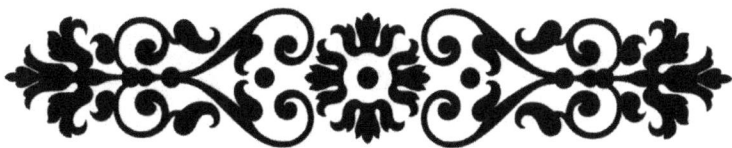

Notes

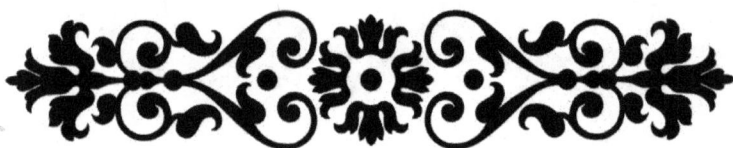

Notes

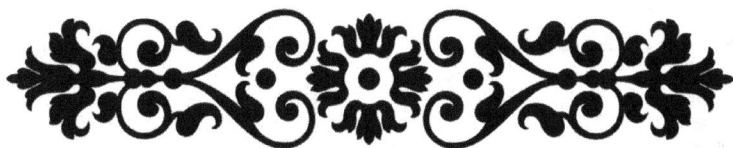

Notes

Bibliography

Many of the ideas contained within have had their foundation in the books I have listed below. Each book is full of invaluable information and I highly recommend you read them at your leisure separately.

Eckhart Tolle, *A New Earth*, 2008, U.S.A. Penguin Publishing.

Dr. David Perlmutter, 2015, *Brain Maker*, Great Britain, Yellow Kite Publishing.

Dr. Joseph Mercola, 2015, *Effortless Healing*, U.S.A., Harmony Books.

Liz Wolfe, *Purely Primal Skincare Guide*, 2013, U.S.A., Available as E-book online at http://purelyprimalskincare.com/

Sally Fallon, 2000, *Nourishing Traditions*, U.S.A., New Trends Publishing.

Joshua Rosenthal, 2014, *Integrative Nutrition*, U.S.A., Greenleaf Book Group LLC.

Sarah Ballantyne PhD, 2015, *The Paleo Approach*, U.S.A., Victory Belt Publishing Inc.

Chris Kresser, 2013, *Your Personal Paleo Code*, U.S.A., Little Brown and Company.

Dr. Carole Hungerford, 2006, *Good Health in the 21st Century*, Australia, Scribe.

References

[i] Aus. Bureau of Statistics, last accessed 4 June 2016,
http://www.abs.gov.au/ausstats/abs

[ii] Aus. Institute of Health and Welfare, last accessed 4 June 2016
http://www.aihw.gov.au/australias-health/2014/ill-health/

[iii] Aus. Bureau of Statistics, last accessed 4 June 2016
http://www.abs.gov.au/ausstats/abs

[iv] World Health Organization Cancer Fact Sheet, updated Feb 2015, last
accessed 4 June 2016 http://www.who.int/mediacentre/factsheets

[v] American Autoimmune Related Diseases Association, Inc., Fact Sheet, last
accessed 4 June 2016, http://www.aarda.org/autoimmune-
information/autoimmune-statistics/

[vi] Bruce Lipton, 2015, *The Biology of Belief*, U.S.A. Hay House Inc.

[vii] Mayo Clinic, last accessed 4 June 2016, http://www.mayoclinic.org/healthy-
lifestyle/nutrition-and-healthy-eating/in-depth/water/art-20044256?pg=2

[viii] Mayo Clinic, last accessed 4 June
2016,http://www.mayoclinic.org/diseases-
conditions/dehydration/basics/symptoms/con-20030056

[ix] Malin and Till, 2015, Biomed Central, last accessed 4 June 2016,
http://ehjournal.biomedcentral.com/articles/10.1186/s12940-015-0003-1

[x] Peckham, Lowery, Spencer, 2015, Journal of Epidemiology and Community
Health, last accessed 4 June 2016 http://fluoridealert.org/wp-
content/uploads/peckham-2015.pdf

[xi] National Research Council, 2006, Fluoride's Neurotoxicity and
Neurobehavioural Effects, Fluoride Action Network, last accessed 4 June 2016,
http://fluoridealert.org/studies/brain06/

[xii] http://www.health.gov.au/internet/main/publishing.nsf/content/health-pubhlth-strateg-phys-act-guidelines#apaadult

[xiii] Xie et al "Sleep initiated fluid flux drives metabolite clearance from the adult brain." *Science*, October 18, 2013. DOI: 10.1126/science.1241224

[xiv] Poulain M.; Pes G.M.; Grasland C.; Carru C.; Ferucci L.; Baggio G.; Franceschi C.; Deiana L. (2004). "Identification of a Geographic Area Characterized by Extreme Longevity in the Sardinia Island: the AKEA study". Experimental Gerontology **39** (9): 1423–1429.*doi:10.1016/j.exger.2004.06.016*. *PMID 15489066*.

[xv] http://www.ncbi.nlm.nih.gov/pmc/articles/PMC3265077/

www.ingramcontent.com/pod-product-compliance
Lightning Source LLC
Chambersburg PA
CBHW060904280326
41934CB00007B/1174